The Revolution Is You!

Your 6-Step Method for a Happier Mind, Healthier Life and Unlimited Results!

I0429440

JASON LEENAARTS

Introduction: A Short(er) Version of a Long(er) Truth

How do I write to inspire? My father wrote those very same words to me about 20 years ago. They have resonated ever since. I've been giving people fitness advice for about 16 years, long before I knew exactly what I was talking about. My path has been far from ordinary and I hope that my background can show you that anyone can turn their life around.

Unlike a lot of other personal trainers, I didn't have an athletic upbringing. I also never had to transform my life from being overweight to someone who got in shape. My transformation journey began when I was still fighting drug addiction.

It wasn't just drugs though. I've been sexually abused, hospitalized multiple times for suicide attempts and suicidal ideation, and over-medicated for illnesses I didn't actually have. When the pharmaceutical drugs failed to provide the relief I wanted, I transitioned to street drugs. On multiple occasions, I've managed to dodge death and incarceration. Despite my parents best efforts to raise me well, there was a side of me that didn't appreciate any level of self control.

Thankfully, I was able to turn things around for myself. It was never easy and it didn't come quickly. I spent ten years addicted to drugs and fitness was the light at the end of the tunnel for me. Even after I found some relief with exercise, it would take a few more years before I got my diet under control, and a few more years still before I would clean up and get off drugs altogether.

My journey wasn't normal and I don't wish my past on anyone. Rather than spend a lot of time hashing out the gory details I want you to appreciate that we all have a battle we've been fighting.

I opened Revolution Fitness and Therapy (RevFit) in the spring of 2009. Since then, we've helped hundreds of clients gain a better understanding of how to change their lives for the better. This book was written with the express interest of taking my story along with the stories of our clients in helping you succeed.

I dedicate this book to several people who inspired its writing. To my father, who lost his battle to multiple myeloma (bone marrow cancer) in 2011. You continue to be the footsteps I aim to follow. To my mother, who survived her own battle with cancer and continues to work with muscular dystrophy, never allowing it to slow her down. Not only do you inspire me but you help keep the voice of my father alive. To my son, Jackson, who remains such a radiant light in my life. Jackson continues to show me that despite his diagnosis of autism, there is nothing that can stand in his way. And last but not least, to my wife, Marissa, for keeping me focused, constantly improving, and driven for more. My love to all of you.

Jason Leenaarts

January 2016

Acknowledgments

I'd like to take a moment to thank Patrick Dahdal of Transformation Publishing for reaching out to me and kickstarting this project. My cousin, Meaghan Beasley, who took time out of her busy schedule to edit my ramblings and pull me into more cohesive thought. Justin Rice, who assisted with photography and formatting of the book itself. Nate Mannan, who designed the book cover and gave my ideas some life. And of course, all of my clients, past and current whose experiences, struggles, successes and stories inspired the completion of this book. Your lives and your contributions are invaluable.

How to Approach This Book

Over the past six years, I have been honored to work with hundreds of clients who wanted to make a change. Many came to me with the goal of weight loss, while some just needed to be held accountable for their goals and maintain a better wellness balance. As you can imagine, personalities differ greatly from person to person; so my tactics have developed an ebb and flow to accommodate different people.

My intention with this book is to offer six phases of change. While all should be considered and acknowledged, anyone who reads this book will be working from a different starting place. I'm offering strategies and tactics from essentially two different viewpoints: One approach entails heavy-handed, call-to-action strategies, while the other is soft-handed in comparison. Each tactic will speak to each person differently. You may find that some of what I discuss pinpoints your exact obstacles while other approaches may have little to do with how your life currently operates.

You may find that as you remove obstacles from your life, you may need to return to this book as a reference point.Your philosophy and ability to handle what comes your way shifts as well. As I've told my clients, sometimes we work with Plan A until it no longer proves effective. Then we shift to Plan B, or skip to E!

One of the most important things I hope to teach, is the ability to be flexible. Life will always find a way of disrupting your best intentions. This is to be expected. If we didn't have deviations from the journey, we wouldn't be able to appreciate the changes and nuances of the scenery!

If you allow your mind to accept the bumps along the way, you have greater potential not only for change but for results that you can sustain. After reading about my background in the introduction, you know I had to take many hard and uncomfortable looks at myself and my life before I was ready for change. If I had not done so, I would have been doomed to repeat many of the destructive behaviors that defined parts of my life.

Mind you, I'm far from perfect and the goal of perfection was never mine to chase. I needed progress and I needed to be able to look back and say, "Wow, I achieved that."

Most of what you'll read here has been based on what I've used and seen succeed for my clients. Ultimately, I want you to know that many people share similar stories to your own. I hope these approaches resonate and provoke change for you.

I'll discuss this in further detail soon, but your success in how you approach this book is purely dependent on your desires. Many people consider their current situation as a "need" to change. Needs are great and all, but I've found that far more can be accomplished when a sincere and burning "want" can overpower the "need."

Phase 1-Your Mind

Why Mindset Matters

Some things should just come easily. If you start a diet, it should be simple to follow. If you start exercising, there should be immediate benefits and results since you're working up a sweat. What you may find as we go through this process is that the steps are simple in theory but not necessarily easy to implement. This is where your mind or, more appropriately, your mindset will help you.

I'm a big believer in telling yourself things that inspire confidence. We are all motivated differently. Some people need to see an image on social media telling us to push harder or give it your all; such as a photo of a very fit individual dripping with sweat and achieving the goals we hope to. Others need to be shown the error of their ways to influence change. The key to your success is not only telling yourself that you "can" but asking yourself if you "will."

The problem with mindset can be a bit like the problem with willpower, sometimes it just isn't there or, if it is there, it's not firing on all cylinders. Some of the most optimistic people I know have down days, just like some of the most depressed and negative people I know have days where it seems the sun actually shines in their direction.

Without giving you some fluffy, zen-like answer to your mindset woes, I'd like to help guide you to places you might not normally take yourself.

Ask yourself what really matters to you. Is it...

Weight loss? Acceptance from others? More energy when you play with your children? To fit into those great jeans you bought a few years ago that you only got to wear a handful of times?

Next determine, what's so important about those goals. How does your life improve if you reach them? Will you automatically have the life of your wishes when you hit your respective goal?

Maybe so.

Probably not.

So where do you start?

Start with being uncomfortable.

"If you wanna learn, get ready to feel dumb nearly all the time. The concepts that make you smarter will be at your border of understanding; exactly where you feel lost. If you wanna get strong, get ready to feel weak a lot. Pushing your physiology hard enough to improve it creates the very fatigue that makes you feel crushed... If you always need to feel smart, strong, and capable, you're not getting as good as you could be, no matter what you think you're doing."-Dr. Mike Israetel

To get anywhere near your fitness, diet, and life you'll need to be comfortable getting uncomfortable. Granted, some things might come easier than others. You might have a natural strength that makes lifting weights not seem as challenging for you. Someone else may be able to dial in their diet and keep their eating on track better than the next.

Somewhere along your journey, you're going to hit a plateau or you're going to fall off the food wagon because things weren't quite in sync. This is where things get uncomfortable. Will you revert to your old ways (the easier path) or modify what you need to keep changing (the harder path)? Old habits will want to creep in and it's your job to keep that door closed.

One of my clients, Don, lost nearly 90 pounds a few years ago while working with me. The weight came off in less than a year. I'm not sure he hit a single sticking point while he was losing the weight. At his lowest, he was only 10 pounds or so away from his dream weight. Around that time, his house flooded. He and his wife had to move into a hotel for a few months until they could get back into their home. While they were there, some of Don's old habits started to rear their heads. One of Don's weaknesses was Coke. As he re-introduced Coke into his drinking regimen, he returned to some old eating habits. Slowly, the weight started coming back. Even after he moved back into his home, Don couldn't distance himself from his drink of choice. In about as much time as it took for him to lose the weight initially, he gained it all back. Why? Mindset.

The good news is that Don is back on the weight loss wagon. We started from the top and said that Coke had to be eliminated. Now, I'm not one of those people who shames certain foods or stands on a soapbox talking about how terrible certain things are for people's health, but Don had some dietary weaknesses that had to be eliminated completely in order to be conquered. Not everyone is like this, but your mindset determines how these things can affect you.

Consider this: what if everything that went wrong in your life was actually your fault? So many people want to point a finger in someone's direction and say "They did this to me" or "It's their fault that I have this problem." Why let someone else take away your power? Own what happens to you so you can work to change it.

Take the example I provided in the introduction about being sexually abused. I didn't do anything wrong per se in that situation but I allowed it to take charge over my life and my feelings. I couldn't come to terms with the fact that a traumatic event happened to me, or that I knew how to overcome it and make myself stronger as a result of it. This in no way meant to trivialize what happened. Sexual abuse of any nature is one of the worst things I can imagine for someone to experience.

I used different avenues to conquer my emotions and

my depression. I wrote about the abuse in poems, I gave speeches about it to raise awareness about sexual abuse. At one point, when I was in college, I even worked up the nerve to call my abuser (13 years after the fact) and confront him about it. Sadly, he had no recollection of the event. The memory and details I provided him were unmistakable. He knew there were things that couldn't be disputed regardless of his own memory of that day. Knowing that I could put that situation behind me gave me closure I couldn't imagine.

"Mindset-A fixed mental attitude or disposition that predetermines a person's responses to and interpretations of situations."

I needed to start this book with mindset for one simple reason: without it, you will likely fail. Your mindset will determine how you perceive every phase of this book. I don't want to get too far ahead of myself right from the get-go, it's not realistic to think that you're going to be 100% driven, committed and on pace the whole way through your journey. You probably won't. But your mindset will determine how quickly you can get back on plan after the deviations.

In conversations with drug addicts, it is called "rock bottom." Rock bottom is where you decide you can't fall any further. I use the same term with people trying to lose weight. For me, that was when I realized that I always had money for drugs but struggled to make my mortgage.

This is where you should appreciate your own stance on what motivates you. I've heard profound reasons and superficial ones. There is no wrong, there is only what keeps you on the path.

From a fitness standpoint, mindset determines if you do one extra rep OR if you even show up to the gym at all. From a diet standpoint, it's the food you eat OR don't eat. In the war with your emotions and stress, it's what you choose to control OR what you allow to control you.

Sounds simple, but it's not.

The fact of the matter is, diet and exercise have come pretty easily for me. I don't find it particularly difficult to adhere to either. Then again, I own a fitness studio so if I couldn't find the time to exercise, I would need to reevaluate the way I manage my time. My struggle lies with financial responsibility, which is something that has taken me an excruciatingly long time to improve. I've used my mindset to improve my financial responsibility in a fairly straightforward way: I run a business with two employees, I have a wife, a son, and a home. If I choose to be financially irresponsible now, the stakes are so high I would stand to lose everything. For those of you who may operate counter to me, many people I know do just fine with their finances but they're all over the map with food and exercise. We all prioritize things differently depending on how they affect us.

How Important is the Placebo Effect?

It would be difficult for me to overestimate the power of a placebo when it comes to how you believe your journey will go. Consider this fascinating example: Most of us have had a headache at one time or another. Different people have different default painkillers that they turn to for relief. Almost immediately, they feel better but it's the placebo effect: the belief that by taking our preferred painkiller we will feel better generally before our body has even broken the medication down. In some clinical trials, the placebo outperforms the actual medication being tested. This doesn't just apply to pain medications but some antidepressants as well.

Imagine being told you're taking part in a trial to help you with your depression. You will be testing a new medication to relieve or minimize your symptoms; instead of receiving the new pill, you receive a sugar pill instead. Because you believe you are taking a medication, within days you note a significant change in your mood, your sleep patterns, and your outlook on life. Clearly, your mind is your most powerful asset.

If you believe you can be successful at weight loss and keeping it off, you stand a better chance of achieving your goal. If you tell yourself that, despite your best efforts, you will probably end up disappointed again then your actions and your beliefs will guide you to that inevitable outcome.

I've found it fascinating how many people I've had the opportunity to coach and counsel who take this very grim and bleak look at their journey:

"Oh, I've tried that. It didn't work."

"That worked okay for me but I gained all the weight back."

"I've basically assumed I'm always going to be at this undesirable weight."

"I thought I'd give this a try but I just don't have very

good luck with getting my weight to budge."

Consider all of this from another perspective. My son, Jackson, is from my first marriage. My first marriage did not end on great terms. Had I approached my second marriage as, "Well, my first one didn't turn out well. This is probably going to be doomed too," then guess what? I'd probably be headed the same direction now. But luckily, Marissa and I are happily married.

While this all pertains to your respective mindset, it's important to realize how vital your expectations of your experience can shape your outcomes. One way to start reshaping how you think is to write about it.

For many of my clients, by the time they walk through my door, they have hit their rock bottom. They don't like what they see in the mirror. Maybe they get out of breath going up and down the stairs. If they've been propelled by the aforementioned thought process of feeling like they can't make progress, it's easy to stay in that downward spiral.

I ask many of them to start making a list of the victories. It doesn't matter if the list is compiled in the note section of their smartphones or written by pen on paper. What matters is that you can add up the small accomplishments that bring you closer not only to your goals but to a more stable belief of what you can do.

We'll talk more about what you document when we start talking about diet and exercise. For now, consider something that allows one success to build on another. It may look something like this:

November 1: Made it to the gym for my first workout. Didn't die!

November 2: Was sore from my first workout but still took the dog for a couple of laps around my neighborhood.

November 3: Made it to the gym for my second workout. Tried a new exercise!

November 4: Started drinking more water and less soda.

November 5: Made it to the gym for my third workout. Someone complimented my efforts and consistency. I didn't think anyone would notice!

I know what you might be thinking; maybe you're a bit more of a self-starter and this is too rudimentary for where you currently stand with your outlook and plan. I'll use myself as an example, since I would be potentially further along than the person in the example above.

Let's assume that while I've been pretty good with diet and exercise, I want a more positive outlook about what I can achieve:

November 1: Started counting calories and using measuring cups to get food in line.

November 2: Ran 1/4 mile further than I had before on my training run.

November 3: Got a full 8 hours of sleep and feel great!

November 4: Was able to lift 5lbs more than I was a month ago on my deadlift.

November 5: Decreased caffeine intake and increased water intake.

The goal is to establish an indisputable trail of progress. It doesn't matter as much WHAT you're doing as long as you're documenting THAT it was done. When you hit those inevitable plateaus, you'll be able to look back at your journal and see what kind of progress you made. This can be far more effective than criticizing yourself for what you didn't do or, maybe, didn't do as well as you might have liked.

In many cases, if we don't have documentation of accomplishments, it's easy to forget how far we've come. It's in those moments of weakness that we can stray from the plan and derail our efforts. This can be especially powerful for those who are working hard to lose weight but not seeing the reflection on the scale.

Smaller Steps, Greater Adherence

Let's talk about your habits: good, bad or otherwise. Whether you're a highly regimented person or you work at a high level of chronic chaos, you've got habits. A regimented person may have many habits and routines that keep them in line with their life. A person who lives in chaos may only allow a few routines to guide them. Wherever you fall on this spectrum, there is always room to improve.

When I start a consultation with a client, there is usually an overview of medical history, injury history, a rough idea of what a daily diet might look like, etc. We also cover goals: weight loss, weight maintenance, weight gain, strength increase, etc. Based on the information I pull together in this session, I can make a general list of changes that should be considered in order to reach the goal.

Normally, this list looks easy to follow. It might be something along these lines:

Increase water intake to 100 oz. per day

Decrease alcohol intake to 1-2 drinks once a week

Exercise 3-4 times a week

Eat less junk food

Start a food journal

Looking at a hypothetical list like this, many of these changes seem very simple to make; however, you may be coming from a different starting place. We all have fairly different lifestyles with different habits that have become ingrained in our day-to-day life. The most effective route to positive change is the one that not enough people attempt to make. Assuming the aforementioned list has the changes it would take for one to reach his/her goals, pick the habit/change that would be the easiest one to make right now.

Just one.

Ask yourself if you believe you have a 90-100% chance of adhering to the change you choose as the most important. If the answer is "yes" then begin there. Focus on that change and that change alone for approximately two weeks, then see what else you can attack on the list.

Unfortunately, many people try to make 2-3 changes immediately. It seems reasonable. "Sure, I can increase water AND decrease alcohol, no problem." It CAN be a problem. In his excellent book, *The Power of Less,* author Leo Babauta notes, "In my experience there is a 100 percent failure rate for forming multiple habits at once, and a 50 to 80 percent rate of success if you do just one habit at a time..."

I have seen some exceptions to this but they are not the norm. I would quantify less than 10% of people can make more radical changes than that and make them stick. That statement is based purely on what I have seen happen with my clients. For all intents and purposes, it may serve you better to assume you are more the rule than the exception.

Let's discuss what happens if the first change you make doesn't stick? There are a couple of approaches you can consider. You may have underestimated the difficulty of the change respective of where your life is currently. If so, you can opt to go back through the list and tackle a different habit. The other option is to scale the change down. For instance, it might be ideal for you to exercise

3-4 times a week but with your current schedule, you can only fit in two workouts a week. This is still a good option, but realize that while the change is heading in the right direction, you may not see results quite as quickly this way. If you're trying to make a lot of changes, it's more effective to start taking baby steps in the right direction as opposed to giant leaps that don't stick and force you into a place where you're doing nothing to advance yourself.

Many of us have patterns and behaviors that are so ingrained in our lives that radical change can leave us discouraged and unwilling to move forward. Rather than dedicating ourselves to the program, we take the first opportunity to deviate and stray off course. In this industry, I tend to hear the adage "It's about the journey, not the destination" or "You're in for the marathon, not the sprint." Whichever statement resonates with you, they both say essentially the same thing: The idea of longevity that you envision for yourself should include a realistic outlook on how you approach:

-Your fitness.

-Your food plan.

-How effectively you can reach and maintain your results.

Think About the Want

Years ago, when I was working part-time at a gym, a gentleman came in to sign up for a membership. He looked like he had been crying. He proceeded to tell the person at the front desk that he needed to get signed up immediately and that he needed a personal trainer. They set him up with one of my co-workers and I happened to be privy to their first conversation together.

The gentleman was crying because he just left his doctor's office who told him that his Type II diabetes was out of control. If he didn't lose weight soon, he would likely need his leg amputated in less than a year. This was enough to scare him straight and he rushed over to the gym to get started. My colleague was kind enough to listen with an sympathetic ear and let him know he was in good hands.

They started training together and every time I worked, I saw this guy come in and get a great workout. In less than a month, he gave up, no more personal trainer. Then his gym attendance dropped down. And just like that he was gone.

One thing I know for sure: if I were faced with losing a limb or part of a limb, and it was within my power to change that outcome, I would move mountains to do so. I've never walked a mile in anyone's shoes but my own so I can't comprehend the battles of someone else. I hope that outside of my field of vision this guy was able to lose weight on his own terms and didn't give up on himself.

The reason I mention this story is almost purely

about semantics. A lot of people say they "need" to lose weight. Like they "need" to save more and spend less or they "need" to get their life in order. It makes perfect sense and that need probably is sincere. What I've found is that the people who tend to succeed at any of these things are the people who want the change, not the people who "need" it.

In my past struggle with financial responsibility, my father used to say that money would burn a hole in my pocket. It wasn't necessarily the fault of my parents. They were both very responsible with their money and my Dad definitely tried to impress that upon me. I have always leaned more towards the impulsive side of things in many areas of my life, much of which I have already shared with you. It took me hitting that point in my life where I wanted more for myself. I knew I had worked hard and I felt as if there should be more to show for it than what I had.

It's important to establish what your want is so the

desire burns bright. I don't want to leave the "need" out of the conversation though. Mary, one of our clients at RevFit, recently stopped smoking. I asked her if she needed to quit or she wanted to. Without hesitation she said, 'I needed to stop. My kids hated it. My son, who is expecting his first baby, flat out told me, Mom, I'm not letting you babysit if you're still a smoker. That was the final straw. I had always wanted to quit, but I don't go half-way with things. I wanted to quit smoking so I could have time with my grandchild."

Ultimately, you need that constant fire to push you towards progress. Define it and determine how it should be constant to keep you honest with yourself.

Exorcising the Demons

I know not everyone has experienced the same back story as me. Many have led relatively calm lives in comparison. As I've delved deeper into what many of my clients have gone through, there are always barriers to success. For some it can be eating disorders, body image issues (a.k.a. Body Dysmorphic Disorder), abusive pasts, addictive behaviors, divorce, death of a loved one, etc. How we manage to cope with any of these things can determine what level of success we ultimately find.

Since I'm no psychologist, I can offer this suggestion: Confront everything you can that might be holding you back from your respective success. Any traumas or stresses can be detrimental to you when it comes to helping you reach your goals. While I can appreciate some level of self-deprecating humor when people talk about themselves, having a sense of self-confidence is imperative if you not only want to reach your goals but maintain them once you've succeeded. This goes back to the conversation on mindset.

When it comes to what you want to achieve both physically and mentally, it helps to take inventory of how you might be potentially sabotaging your efforts. For me, it took therapy, medication, a lot of self-destructive behavior, and, quite honestly, a great deal of trial and error to stubbornly stumble through a path to success. Now that I've found that proverbial light at the end of the tunnel, it's about carving new paths along the way.

It's also worth noting that we essentially determine our own destiny. It would have been somewhat easy for me to look at my life and play the victim to my own circumstances:

Because I was sexually abused, my life is forever tainted.

Because I was a drug addict, I'll never find true strength or independence.

Because I was divorced, I'll never find a good relationship or someone to   love me the way I want.

I see divorcees who blame their circumstances purely on how their former spouses treated them. I see employees of corporations who swear their bosses are only out to get them. Maybe they're right, maybe it's the wrong place to work and they need to be somewhere that upper management can appreciate their skills and give them room to grow. A great deal of our outcomes stem from allowing disruptive patterns to take over without breaking them.

Your life is about your choice. There will be things that spiral out of your control, this is true. Adopting an approach that allows you to look at what you're capable of controlling makes the obstacles much easier to overcome. I wasn't going to allow myself to be defined by my past. Most of it is ugly, some of it was wonderful. All of it helped me gain a better understanding of how I could change and improve myself. Since I opened my business, I've spent thousands of hours (and dollars) on self-improvement. The way I see it, that journey will never (and should never) end.

If I can accomplish anything with this book, I'd like to see if I can save you thousands of dollars in self-improvement. Chances are, you may have already spent that money over the years searching for a solution.

What I can promise you is that you will definitely spend thousands of hours in self-improvement, as you should. It isn't intended to be a quick fix. There is no pill. In the next several phases of the book, I'm going to help you take inventory of things in your life. Some will be obvious, some less so.

I will say that whatever you think is standing in your way, it needs to be addressed. Sometimes you can talk it over with a spouse or significant other. Sometimes it may take the help of a qualified therapist or psychiatrist. It took 5 different psychiatrists before I found the one who solved my riddle and saved my life. You may be lucky enough to find the right fit for you with greater ease than I did.

Allow this book to offer solutions and perspective.

Phase I Action Plan

1. Ask yourself if this is the right time to make changes in your life. Consider the obstacles (family, work, current schedule) that might be standing in the way of your progress. What can be removed or modified?

2. Remember that your outlook on how you move forward has a direct correlation with the level of your success. Start taking notes about what positive things you're going to do (or have done) to get yourself closer to where you want to be.

3. Make a list of the changes you believe you need to make to get your body where you want. Start the list now and be prepared to add more to it as you work your way through this book.

4. Ask yourself: What change can I make with almost 100% commitment right now? Start with that change and stick to it until it feels natural and automatic. Only then do you move to the next change.

5. Confront your fears and hesitations. Write them out if you have to. Be honest with yourself about past experiences, doubts and concerns. Make sure these things are not standing in the way of your ability to make progress.

Phase II-Your Environment

The Workplace

Consider how your job and potentially just the workplace itself creates unnecessary stress for you. Toxic co-workers, condescending boss, unreasonable deadlines, messy desk, no room for advancement without making a deal with the devil first, the list can go on.

Now, you can certainly go the route I went and turn in your resignation to a perfectly good salary. I don't recommend it but it did work for me. Or you can look at what things you actually have the influence to change.

Look at your desk. Is it messy? Stacks of files and paperwork everywhere? Coffee mugs with days old coffee that didn't get washed out? Snack wrappers on the floor from your attempts at reliving your high school basketball days?

Clean it. Seriously. Right now.

Years ago, I worked for a pretty unsavory guy. This man had no qualms about rushing in during the middle of a work day and cussing you out right in front of the customers. He was great like that.

However, like many situations, there was a positive to pull from my experience under him. He not only taught me what kind of supervisor I didn't want to be, he gave me a lesson that has stuck with me for nearly 20 years.

One afternoon, he surprised us with a visit. We were handling inventory at our sales counter, a common practice while we were stocking our shelves. He came right in, made a beeline for the register and asked, "You know what I hate?" I offered a blank stare, waiting for my next reaming. "I hate a dirty kitchen. NO ONE wants to cook in a dirty kitchen. So you know what we're going to do? We're going to clean our kitchen before we start cooking!" Mind you, we weren't in a kitchen but I caught his drift.

Sometimes, it takes someone breathing down your neck to see things in just the right light.

So, I offer you the same lesson: look at your desk. Is your kitchen dirty? Clean it. The clutter, which may seem somewhat organized to you is taking up not only physical space but mental space as well. It's blocking your vision. It's keeping you from breathing. Does it need to be so clean you could eat off it? Not necessarily, but it wouldn't hurt.

File your paperwork, clean your mugs, give yourself a clear point of view. Straighten the photos of the spouse and kids. Maybe you should frame them instead of sticking push pins through them. Give your space some much needed love. Now, stand back and admire your handiwork. To what degree disorganization gives you stress is debatable, but organization can eliminate the stress. Take control of what you can. If you can't control your boss, control your area. If you can't control your co-workers, control yourself. There are VERY few areas of your life you have complete and total control over. This is one of those few things. Handle it. Embrace it. Clean it. NOW you're ready to cook.

What if you're one of those who keeps your area immaculate? My hat's off to you. Keep it that way so others have a leader to follow.

Now, how about that email?

That's right: look at your inbox, your subfolders, all of those things filed away which may or may never be accessed again.

What can you delete? Any old coupons or discounts from retail mailing lists which have expired? Do you really need to be on those lists anyway? Start unsubscribing from places you don't utilize often enough for it to have any bearing on your life. Every retailer and professional in the nation has a mailing list. I'm no exception. Some of these businesses and business professionals are kind enough to email you once every two weeks. Some email you EVERY SINGLE DAY. That's obnoxious. Unsubscribe.

What you're doing to your inbox is similar to what you did for your desk, removing the clutter. Even if you're good about deleting your emails regularly and responding to all requests within 24 hours, your subfolders can be housing hundreds (maybe thousands) of things you don't really need. It's time to spring clean (even if it's winter).

How about the breakroom? What do you have access to? Processed snacks, vending machines, donuts from a sales rep who was trying to make an impression? If you can't remove the less healthy options, see if you can add some better ones. Ask someone if a fruit bowl can be made available. Many fruits can be available for a week or so before they go bad. Offer to supply the fruit for reimbursement. You need better selections.

Worst case, keep some choices at your own desk. If

that's the first visible option, you're removing temptation. Keep snack bags of nuts or jerky in your desk for when you're craving something. In most cases, 20-24 almonds will do the trick but make sure they're in their respective bags. Don't tear into a jar of them and expect that you can moderate the amount. Many people cannot.

Why the big fuss over the workplace? Because this is where you spend upwards of 40 hours a week, maybe more. That's almost 25% of the time in a week. If you allow the things which are under your control to spiral out in a place that you give that much of your time to, I can tell you which side is winning and your side isn't looking favorable.

The Home

There is just one way to escape this negative spiral—by tidying efficiently all at once, as quickly as possible, to make the perfect clutter-free environment. – The Life Changing Magic of Tidying Up, Marie Kondo

In her book, *The Life Changing Magic of Tidying Up,* Marie Kondo outlines the principles for removing clutter from your life. While she primarily discusses this with regard to your home, you may find some of her philsophies can apply to the workplace as well. If you walk into a mess when you get home, cleaning it can either become a priority over other things or you can continue to live with the mess.

That being said, you have vastly more control over how your house looks than the place you work. Band together with everyone in your home to establish some rhyme and reason. Delegate tasks, get rid of the non-essentials.

It might seem trite but simple tasks like making sure the bed is made, wiping down your bathroom counters, toilets, etc. can be immensely effective at giving you a sense of accomplishment and productivity. I'll be the first to admit, dust doesn't always catch my attention but clutter absolutely does.

Everyone has a different barometer for what they can reasonably deal with. There will always be the exceptions to the rule who function well-surrounded in little messes. I don't know many like this but they do exist.

You might be wondering why I'm putting so much emphasis on cleanliness. It isn't because I have some obsessive trait that makes it unbearable. However, there is a direct link between clutter and stress as well as clutter and depression. Keeping up with how your home and office look is basically just taking care of low-hanging fruit. It's easy to manage and an easy problem to solve. If you get the extra added bonus of less stress and potentially less depression it becomes a win-win.

"Clutter bombards our minds with excessive stimuli (visual, olfactory, tactile), causing our senses to work overtime on stimuli that aren't necessary or important."-Dr. Sherrie Carter

By doing some of these things that seem somewhat out of the realm of "health and fitness," you're giving yourself fewer obstacles to hurdle when it comes time to focus on the things that seem more obvious. It's these factors that sit in our periphery that can help establish some sense of order to your life. As you start to stack more of these positives in the right direction, you'll find that when the conversation changes to food and exercise, much of the other obstacles are out of your way and dealt with. Throughout the book, we'll continually be searching for the path of least resistance in your life.

Let's move forward with the rest of the "housekeeping."

Social Media and More

I recently heard the results of a study stating that the average smartphone user checks their phone 110 times a day. That's incredible. Now, more than ever, we're completely glued to our phones. We have instant access to information, entertainment, personal contacts, our appointments and more. No matter where you stand with your opinion of them, for the foreseeable future, smartphone use and the dependency on electronic devices is here to stay.

This brings me to the last part of the environmental section. For as great as the web is for giving us information, we are completely bombarded by polarizing views and hypersensitive people. I frequently check my Facebook pages and it never ceases to amaze me how much negativity is on broadcast for all to see. On any given day, liberals slam conservatives, conservatives slam liberals, one type of parent shames another for the way they raise their children, the list goes on.

Some do a great job of not allowing this stimulus to affect them. I find it permeates the way I think and feel. I literally have to unfollow certain people I connect to because the things they have to say are completely unproductive and they don't help me further my life.

Those who are able to avoid the lure of Facebook, Twitter, etc. are still affected by the bias of many news outlets, spam emails in their inbox, and television as well. It becomes difficult to steer clear of the influences we're exposed to.

So before we start shifting our focus to the people who are directly involved in our lives, the last things I want to mention to you in regards to environmental stressors are about this electronic influence.

I'm a big fan of music, always have been. I'm always on the lookout for new bands or artists to listen to. As a result, much of what is in my Facebook feed is music based. However, periodically I have to go through to unlike and unfollow certain pages. I have to be realistic with myself and ask if I still need to actively follow everyone that I do. It ends up becoming too much to sift through when I want to be engaged on Facebook. Not to mention, it starts a snowball effect of getting lost in pages of News Feed just to feel like I can be a part of what's there.

In addition, if you've ever tried to get serious about getting your food and exercise in order, it's easy to accumulate stacks of pages to follow telling you to eat this way or that, or to train one way or another. If that's the case, you're already well aware of the fact that opinions fall on opposite ends of the spectrum for both! I recently signed up a client who told me specifically that one of the reasons he hired me was because he was so sick of seeing opposing views on food and fitness all over the internet.

There will always be a keyboard warrior who stands contrary to what you've been told or led to believe. It's people like this who make us second guess ourselves and not stick to a given program. For the same reason that you should not gauge your level of success on what you see your neighbor do, you should also steer clear of the same advice towards Anonymous1234 who says they got a great body from that new fitness gadget they purchased from an infomercial!

Just like I've encouraged you to remove and organize clutter in your work and in your home, it's time to do the same with social media. Regardless of which avenue you frequent (Facebook, Twitter, Instagram, LinkedIn) they're all potentially time wasters and have to be regulated unless you make a living being active on there. In case you're wondering, most people do not.

It probably speaks volumes to the problem that there are even apps for your phone and your internet browser which allow you to lock certain portions of software and sites so that you're not tempted to browse incessantly and be more unproductive. Time spent actively on things that aren't making you better or getting you closer to your goals are virtual rabbit holes. You can literally chase them and lose hours of a day. Going back to the statistic mentioned above, if you spent 30 seconds every time you checked your phone (sometimes it's less, sometimes it's MUCH more), you would have spent 55 minutes wasting your day!

However, I can be realistic too. Some people need the connection to the outside world. I completely understand. I'm not saying that you have to remove this link from your life, but you still should strive for a less cluttered social media atmosphere as well. Remove games from your phone, delete contacts of people you never intend to call, give yourself time-frames of when you can or can't check email or Facebook if necessary. I know many people who won't even look at their emails until 10am or noon each day. I know others who don't check their email at all on a weekend. Depending on what type of job you do, this may be more or less practical for you.

The bottom line is: it's going to help you in the long run in finding ways to minimize how much stimulation and feedback you get from all sources of media. Anything you can do to de-clutter what you're exposed to will help you in filtering the good from the bad.

Let's tackle the next part: your support system.

Phase II Action Plan

1.) What can you organize at your workplace to make your area less cluttered and more in control? Don't forget to clean not only what's physically there but the "virtual" messes on your computer as well.

2.) Delegate the tasks at your home to everyone living there. Look at things that are more than a year old. Can they be thrown out? Were they even utilized within the last year? If you must hold on to something that doesn't get a lot of use, consider boxing those things up and putting them somewhere out of sight (garage, attic, etc.)

3.) Aim for the same goals with the influences you take from your electronic devices. Unfollow negative people and unsubscribe from mailing lists that don't serve to consistently benefit you. Remove apps and games from your phone or mobile device that are only distracting you from progress and a healthier outlook.

Phase III- Your Support

Your Family

Over the years of training women, men, and children one thing remains firmly planted in my mind: we are all motivated by very different things. In many ways, our family is our front line of defense when it comes to offering support and being there for us through thick and thin. However, the fact that we are motivated in different ways and for different reasons can be problematic for some.

I did not grow up in a family that advocated strength training and regular exercise. Don't get me wrong, it wasn't that we were all a bunch of couch potatoes. In my family, work was the primary activity. There wasn't much time for exercise when you work beyond a standard eight hour day. The window to fit in exercise would close if the work day was closer to 12 hours, leaving a little bit of time for family socializing, dinner and bedtime.

I was the first in my family to start attacking exercise as a regular occurrence. Once the bug bit me, I was basically hooked. Thankfully, my parents saw the positive changes it made for me and they each found a place in which to introduce it for themselves. Since I am an only child, I didn't have any siblings to lead the way in terms of having a headstart with athletics or team sports. In fact, most of my interest in sports died down by time I got to high school.

I've been fortunate to train a lot of families. So many of them work in harmony to support the others in terms of reaching their goals and maintaining a sense of balance in their lives. By the same token, sometimes bad habits can flesh themselves out and negatively affect the outcomes.

It reminds me of a client I've worked with in the past. Diane always struggled a bit with food. She had the same 10-15lbs that she fought to lose. She knew how to train and she knew how to eat. The problem was her husband.

Now, Diane's husband was actually very supportive of her goals; however, he definitely did not need to lose weight. He worked an active job, was naturally very lean and could stockpile junk food with little ill effect. Try as she might to discourage him from bringing candy and treats home, that was what he chose to refuel himself with (in addition to all of their normal meals). Not to mention, many times she would have fed herself appropriately throughout the day, only to join him late at night to eat after she had already eaten what she needed to. Needless to say, weight loss forever became an obstacle for her.

So how do you tackle this?

One way is to have a sincere heart-to-heart with your loved ones. Explain to them the desire to lose weight. Explain your weakness with certain trigger foods. If at all possible, some spouses (like Diane's) should try and eat the trigger foods away from the home. It can be a similar effect to living with a recovering alcoholic. For some, the sight of another drink can send them down the wrong path. Whether you agree with the concept of food addiction or not, if we know that cookies are our downfall and we smell a home-baked chocolate chip cookie, it can be an invitation for disaster.

Another place to be aware of vulnerabilities is with your children. It's not uncommon to have children who can burn through calories like it's nothing. They can eat junk food ad nauseum (pun intended) and never gain a pound. Ah, the luxuries of youth. It also leaves temptation constantly in our faces when the pantry is full of poor quality foods that work great for the kids and not so great for the parents. I've seen time and again how young athletes can consume mountains of calories and never gain an ounce simply because they're so active in their respective sports. However, we as the parents generally don't have the same luxuries!

My challenge to you is to make the journey a team effort. Rally the troops (spouse, kids, significant other, even the dog!) and discuss how you need their help to be successful. Generally speaking, families want to be there for one another. In some cases, a parent AND a child need to work to lose weight. If guidelines can be established to minimize or remove trigger foods from the home, it's a step in the right direction.

It can also be helpful to have a system of rewards that doesn't involve food. Too often, food is used as the gift for a bad day, a good day or a "just because." I'm not saying it isn't a nice gesture but many people use desserts and calorie-laden restaurant choices as the reward for loved ones. This can be terribly counterproductive if all you're trying to do is keep the weight loss going. Between extra calories that get consumed in a moment of weakness and the sodium that gets packed into so many foods, weight can spike up without us even knowing it. Granted, unless you're bound and determined to overindulge, it isn't legitimate weight but extra water weight.

Many of my clients are shocked to hear that a 4lb variance on any given day is 100% normal. That means, that your weight can swing by 4lbs in either direction and be okay! So, it helps to have a realistic sense of what can happen and how your family can help you stay the course.

If children are involved in losing weight too, I have to caution you on using the word "diet" around them. If you're constantly throwing that term around, it can foster eating disorders in minors who don't appreciate the necessity of eating healthier and taking care of their bodies. Sadly, more and more parents are coming to me for help with their minors because of disorders such as bulimia, anorexia, and orthorexia. While I don't have the psychological pedigree to treat these disorders, much of what affects our children is the influence of what they see and hear around them. Never mind the fact that unrealistic Photoshopped images are peeking at them at every magazine stand. They also see their parent(s) struggle with weight issues leading them to believe they need to fall on the opposite extreme of the spectrum to keep from ending up in the same boat.

As opposed to saying that you're going on a diet, change the dynamic of the effort by saying the family needs to focus on a healthier lifestyle. These days, most families have a relative who is battling a lifestyle related challenge: type II diabetes, high blood pressure, high cholesterol, stroke, etc. Any comparison to what other have struggled with within the bloodline can be motivation for a change within your own family.

I'm not going to stand on any soapbox and rehash the difficulties of what these problems can present. The fear of being on medication, which could present another host of side effects, is a big deal for a lot of people. Your family is the foundation for how you can impress and maintain change. To be frank, you (as the parent) are the role model. Whether it's common discussion in the household or not, if you can take control over your health and wellness it can be an infectious change which others can latch onto and utilize as well.

So, where else is this important?

Your Friends

I love my friends. There are people I can go great lengths of time without reaching out to, pick up a phone and we can catch up right where we left off. In my opinion, that's the best kind of friend to have. Due to the amount of hours I work and my very unorthodox working schedule, it doesn't always allow for a proper social life. In addition, it can take away time from my wife or my son and I always try to make sure they get as much of me as possible too.

While our friends can be our best allies when it comes to our wellness goals, they can unfortunately be barriers to our success as well. You see, in many cases, our friends truly want what's best for us. They love seeing us happy and healthy. However, everyone is in a different place with their own journey and sometimes we have those friends who can exhibit a bit of jealousy if we're closer to our goals than they are.

It's not a knock on who we've picked as friends. It's just a common occurrence. One of my nearest and dearest friends, Crissy went through a horrible phase of life when she was diagnosed with thyroid cancer. I was living out of state at the time and was not privy to everything she was going through. We had a mutual friend (we'll call her Kim) who was living closer to Crissy and was able to be a great support. As Crissy was in and out of hospitals being treated for cancer, Kim was there at so many points to be a rock for her. In fact, I'm not sure where Crissy would be if Kim hadn't been such a good friend back then. After Crissy got through the worst of it, she began to regain her strength and confidence in her capacities. At one point when Crissy was essentially in the clear, Kim made the mistake of saying, "You know,

I kind of liked you better when you were sick!"

Now, I've never been in Crissy's shoes, nor have I been in Kim's, but this totally threw Crissy for a loop. This once great friend showed a new set of colors that no one ever really expected. And while this is obviously an extreme case of a friendship gone awry, sometimes our friends don't know how to stay supportive to us when things are both up AND down.

Many of my clients are very social people. They like to party or they're constantly being pulled in different directions for social events. At any point and time, there can be this push-and-pull with our best laid plans for ourselves versus the best wishes of our friends.

This is where things may get a bit delicate. On the one hand, you don't want to turn away good people in your life. On the other hand, you have to remember that your goals are purposefully about your health and longevity. Temporarily, you may have to be particular about the friends you'll associate with if you find they only bring you back to bad habits.

This can accomplish more than one positive. Let's be honest: going out and being social can really put a hit on the finances. Take a nice dinner, some drinks and any other festivities, and the dollars add up quickly. By extending yourself the courtesy of staying in a bit more, you've got more control over what happens with your finances and your waistline.

This doesn't mean you still can't enjoy yourself. You're just being more strategic about the how, when, and who. If you sincerely can't avoid the social outings, there is still a workaround. Try and eat a reasonable meal before you hit the town and drink water frequently to give yourself a greater sense of satiety. This can help you moderate your eating behaviors when you're with your friends.

Most importantly, seek out the friends who genuinely want you to reach your goals. Explain the importance of it. The people in your life with whom this resonates will not only support you throughout the journey, but they'll pull you back to the path if you start to waver, too. Unlike your family, your friends don't have to live with you and that separation can be beneficial when it comes to staying the course.

Your Mentors

I've been very fortunate to have several people in my corner who have been able to help me along the way. While family and friends have their own respective place in my life, the mentors I have had the privilege to work with have been in the position to help steer my focus and either reign me in or help me branch out when needed.

Sometimes family members are too close to give us an unbiased point of view. While they generally have our best interests at heart, being too close to someone emotionally can affect the way we receive criticism and advice; friends are no exception. Mentors, on the other hand, are there in many ways to offer feedback on situations that others may have no experience in. While I do consider my mentors friends as well, there is generally a consensus of a bit less social involvement with them. This isn't exclusive to having a mentor.

I have a doctor friend who I've known almost as long as I've had my business. I trust him with my life. We don't spend a great deal of time together outside of professional settings but I know that if I needed him to be there as a sounding board, he would drop everything to be there for me. He also helps me gain a better understanding of the things I need to tackle professionally. Although we're both health professionals he sees things through a completely different lens than I do. We happen to share some patients/clients together and his insight helps me dive deeper into understanding how to help. I have no hesitation in saying, he's a bit higher up the food chain than I am and I'm not just referring to gross annual income!

Some people like to use catch phrases to describe the mentors in their life. For some it's a mastermind group, for others it's a committee. I challenge you to find people like this who can help you gain some perspective. It may be something as simple as having an accountant and a financial adviser. We need people like this to help remove emotions from the decisions we need to make, people who can help us reach our goals without standing in our way to get there.

Hopefully if you're reading this, you have goals, ambitions, and dreams for yourself. Align yourself with mentors who can help sharpen this focus. As I'm writing this I can think of a small handful of people who I would qualify for this position: two doctors (a chiropractor and an optometrist), an owner of a hair salon/spa, an owner of a massotherapy clinic, a professor of continuing education, and several others who may fluctuate in and out of a given role. These people not only inspire me to be greater, but in my eyes, they have accomplished things that I can't quite fathom, some from a monetary position and some from a position of outlook. All of these people are crucial to my growth.

Consider those in your life might fill these roles. Ask them questions about how they got to where they are in their lives. What were their obstacles, how did they overcome them, and what would they have done differently looking back? How can you apply any of these perspectives to your own life and journey?

And might I add, it's important to continue looking at all of this as a journey. You will have setbacks, you will get discouraged, you will plateau or lose your footing along the way. Look to your mentors to help set you straight again. In my opinion, some of the best conversations I have had with my mentors is when I was able to give a little bit back to them. Sometimes my perspective   is enough to get them to look at their situation in a better light.

So, it's important to have the support you need in life from friends, family and your mentors. Sometimes you'll need to take perspectives from all three and sometimes only one opinion will prevail. Ultimately, as long as you're giving back at least as much as you're receiving, your relationships with your support systems will thrive.

That being said, if you're constantly searching for advice without acting on it, you'll flounder. And if you are the type of person who has a counterargument to every bit of wisdom, you're setting yourself up for failure. There is a hint of success in anything that someone tells you out of care for you. It may not be the best plan of action at the moment but it comes from the right place and should be positively considered.

Truth be told, I sometimes fall into the position of the latter. Because there are so many different things I've done over the years to improve my business, I may hear a bit of advice on something I've tried to do in the past without success. Perhaps the advice didn't work at one point in my career but could work famously now. It doesn't remove the validity of the advice. It may mean I have to find a new way to conquer the same obstacle.

Conventional marketing advice says to test, test and retest. To do so, you have to be ready and willing to fail. By failing, you can have another perspective on what could work with a slightly different tweak and approach.

Ask a lot of questions from your support system. Not everyone is going to know what it's like to be in your shoes. I have a friend who also runs a fitness business a few miles down the road from me. He caters to a slightly different demographic than I do. An elitist point of view might scoff at our relationship and not allow me to interact and learn from a competitor. But I don't view my friend that way. I think there are things we can both learn to be better not just in our businesses but for a better customer experience as well.

So far, we've tackled your mindset, your environment, and your base of support. Some of you may be wondering if the exercise and diet component will be mentioned. It's my belief that the three phases we've discussed so far are every bit as important as your fitness and food. If you can set the stage for your mentality, the area(s) around you, and the people who will stand by your side, the food and fitness will be easier changes to make than you can imagine.

Are you ready for more change?

Phase III Action Plan

1.) Rally the troops!! Talk to your family about the support you feel you need to reach your goals. Have a sincere discussion about how they can benefit from your greater attention to your health as well. Bonus points if you can get a family member to partner up with you.

2.) Look at your friends with the right goal in mind. While you don't want to separate strong bonds, find the friends who can help you the most and keep you steady along the way.

3.) Seek out mentors. If not professionally, find the people who have achieved the goals you're hoping to. Get their advice about what worked for them or what they may have done differently. Apply what you can and discard the rest so you can discover your own path to success. Continue to reach out to these people as they can be crucial to you hitting your goals.

Phase IV-Your Diet

Forget the Absolutes

There is nothing more I'd like than to tell you I have the 100% foolproof diet which will be universally accepted by all of my readers with complete success. Sadly, no such thing exists. The very best tips I'm going to share in this portion of the book are probably going to be very far from glamorous. There will be no special pills, fad diet plans or quick fixes. What you will find will be some direction in trying to navigate through the somewhat murky waters of nutrition.

As we go down this path together, I want you to remove a particular notion about diets and diet advice: forget the absolutes. They are almost nonexistent. Carbs, fats, and proteins all have an important role to play. Truths will not really exist in any particular black-and-white fashion. Most of what you will accomplish resides in a gray area. I will do my best to simplify what's out there so you can look at food in the healthiest light possible and to prepare you for almost any occasion.

Remember that while we are all special individuals in many ways, there are some constants in nutrition to consider and respect. Doing so gives you the greatest chance at getting and keeping your hard earned results.

I'm going to present some options to you that should help you make the best decisions that you can with regard to your approach to food. Some people may need to count calories, some may need to watch eating behaviors, others may do just fine to make some very small tweaks to what they currently do. All approaches are 100% effective...for the right individual. For instance, I love to count calories. I like knowing what I should be shooting for relative to my goals, measuring my portions, etc. It isn't something I feel the need to do all of the time but it does help me gain a fresh perspective on where my food may have deviated off the plan at any given point. That being said, many people would do very poorly to count calories. It presents too much pressure and anxiety for people who already have too much of that in their lives. This is where it's important to respect your personality and what you feel might work for yourself.

With the rage in wearable fitness trackers and calorie apps on our smartphones, it has become easier than ever to track what we eat, when we eat and how we burn it off. Not everyone will go the tech route. Some can see great results simply through adding a pedometer and 10,000 steps a day to their routine. So I'd like to approach each of these concepts somewhat equally so you can decide what will work best for you in your current lifestyle.

Calorie Counting

For those who need black-and-white data, calorie counting may offer some insight. You can use calorie apps on your phone or the algorithms plugged into your wearable trackers. My recommendation is to make sure you plug in relevant information such as: age, gender, height, weight, and level of activity. Find your maintenance calories first; this is how many calories you'll need just to keep your body running at an optimal level on any given day. Be forthright with the portions of food you eat because it helps to measure things like cereal and other starches in the diet. Many people are shocked to see what a true serving size of cereal actually looks like as opposed to what seems right based on the size of the dish. Nuts, nut butters, and cheeses are also places to be aware of true serving sizes as these items are extremely easy to overconsume.

You also need to be mindful of the calories you take in when you drink. Alcohol is certainly a place where calories creep in. Anything you might add to flavor your coffee or tea must also be considered. Not to mention any soft drinks, which are not of the diet variety. I've seen a huge trend in clients who come to me who actually eat fairly well but they consume hundreds of calories in what they put into their coffee on a daily basis. This is an extremely easy fix to not only save calories but your waistline as well!

There are some caveats to calorie counting, though. Calories are not an exact science and even the apps and fitness trackers can have significant margins of error. In addition, eating out at restaurants can present problems because not every restaurant posts their calorie information for the public to see. Restaurants often cook with more oil or butter than what you might expect. This oversight can cause a surplus of hundreds of calories more than what you bargained for.

So, you can use calorie counting for a guideline in trying to understand where you are currently with your eating habits and to see where modifications should be made. It's also important to understand where you should create deficits so you can see weight loss. One approach is to cut your maintenance calories by only 10-15%. This doesn't seem like much but it can create small beneficial changes which will help you lose weight steadily over time. When you add exercise on top of that caloric deficit, the energy expended increases and more weight is then lost.

The problem with many calorie trackers is the weight loss component can be too aggressive for some. When calories are cut too severely, it can cause a host of issues including binge eating, hormone and thyroid disruptions, and poor sleep patterns. While this approach might work for some in the short term, the goal of this book is to give you change that sticks; not the kind of change that makes you resent you ever tried it in the first place. By aiming for sustainable changes, you're setting yourself up for easier adherence and less rebound effect when food becomes unpredictable.

There is another approach to calorie counting which does not require using any particular app or tracker. Very simply put, take your current weight and multiply it by 10-12. This will give you a starting point from which to lose weight. Keep in mind that for this to work optimally, you will need to add activity to your regimen. I will also say that due to the biological differences between men and women, a woman might shoot for a multiple of 10 or 11 while a man may shoot for a multiple of 11 or 12. This is because most men have more muscle than women in proportion to body fat. That increase in muscle can give men an advantage in weight loss when it comes to how quickly results are seen. It's not necessarily fair but that's just the science.

For example, if you're a woman who weighs 150lbs, your calorie goal would be somewhere between 1500 and 1650 per day. If you're a man who weighs 230lbs, your calorie goal would be somewhere between 2530 and 2760 per day. Please note that for any calorie counting protocol, you will need to track your food appropriately to see where you fall in accordance with your goal.

Eating Behaviors

As mentioned above, tracking calories can be a bit intimidating for some. Fortunately, there's another effective way to manage your intake. For busy individuals, another approach can be to watch and document your eating behaviors.

I can't begin to tell you how many parents I train who are busy focused on taking care of their children and spouses while trying to balance their own health as well. It's not hard to imagine many of these people skip meals. Your body is smart and can adapt to almost any deviation in the norm; however, your body needs nutrients to perform and function at an optimal level. Skipping meals might seem like a good way to lose weight but it rarely works.

What typically happens is meals are skipped at the beginning of the day and then people overeat later in the day because they feel so famished. In addition, stress levels can affect people in different ways and cause many to overeat because they're only trying to comfort themselves and not listening appropriately to their body's signals.

One way to change this pattern is to start documenting your eating behaviors. You don't have to show anyone but you do need some proof of what's happened. You can even use the notepad on your smart-phone. What I've found particularly insightful is listing times and food choices. A sample might look something like this:

8am-Coffee with creamer and sugar

1030am-Coffee with creamer and sugar

Noon-Protein bar from gas station

1230pm-Handful of trail mix

4pm-A couple of handfuls of chips

7pm-Salad with dressing, steak, potatoes, and broccoli

8pm-Handful of pretzels

Now, all we did is list times and meal choices. Very little is mentioned about portion size and there is no mention whatsoever about calories. What feedback would I offer a client eating like this who might want to lose weight?

I would ask this client to look at their coffee intake at both intervals in the morning. Can less creamer and sugar be used?

Is water introduced into the day at all?

Also, since a protein bar was convenient at noon, could a protein bar be consumed in the morning to help give a better sense of satiety?

What was happening at 8pm that you felt the need to eat pretzels only an hour after a large dinner? Were you bored, stressed, or actually hungry?

For many people, they've trained their bodies to expect a certain pattern of behaviors. Many feel the need to have dessert or at least something sweet after their dinner to help balance the salty and the sweet. Changing this pattern by removing yourself from the places where food is readily available can help.

I typically will distract myself after a big meal so that I don't take any influence from external cues. For example, if I eat a big meal but I continue to stay close to the kitchen, it's easy to think about other food that I might want to eat...even if I'm full! If I remove myself from the room and find something to occupy my mind, I'm less likely to consider what might be in the cupboard.

One excellent tip I received from a client years ago was for me to floss and brush my teeth immediately after dinner. Since most people have no desire to do this twice, it's a great reminder to steer clear from that extra little snack after dinner!

By examining some of these patterns of behavior for a few days, you could lose weight by changing the way you treat food without counting calories.

Random Dietary Tweaks

There are some other concepts worth considering which might help you as well. As you go through the list, some items will already be on point for you while others may have slipped past you as effective options.

1.) Fill your plate up in each meal like this: half of the plate with green veggies, a quarter of the plate with a starch (rice, corn, potatoes, bread) and the other quarter with a lean protein.

2.) Drink at least half your body weight in ounces of

water per day (no more than a gallon).

3.) For every cup of coffee or tea, drink 10-12 ounces of water.

4.) Reduce alcohol intake to once per week and no more than two servings (at a time).

5.) Try a new vegetable every week.

6.) Take your largest meal of any given day and cut the portion in half.

7.) Increase your fiber intake by 5 grams (g) every week. Women should aim for 20-25g a day and men can be closer to 30-35g.

8.) Shoot for no less than 20g of protein every time you eat a meal.

9.) Share your dessert. Challenge yourself to three moderate bites, savoring each one like it's the best dessert you've ever had.

10.) Join or start a recipe club. Get all members to

submit options that are no more than 500 calories per serving. Then start shooting for 300-400 calorie options that might be even more satisfying.

11.) Experiment with spices and herbs instead of condiments: replace mustard, ketchup and mayo with rosemary, black pepper or garlic salt.

These ideas may not seem like much when you read through them but they can spark enough change to get your eating habits headed in the right direction. While some of these concepts may be calorie driven, other concepts give you the flexibility to get creative and look for options which might be more practical for you.

By removing the stress of strict calorie counting or documenting your eating behaviors, you'll be tackling some simple changes which may spark the weight loss you're looking for. Sometimes, the perspective is enough to give you the feeling of significant change.

One last thought with regards to dietary tweaks: make sure you're getting ample protein in each meal. I like to see people shoot for at least 20g per meal, and in many cases, at least 30g for the main meals (breakfast, lunch and dinner.) This can be accomplished with a protein shake, a palm-sized portion of meat/fish or two servings of Greek yogurt. Keep it simple!

It's Okay To Fail

The most common mistake I see people make is allowing their dietary deviations to snowball into complete benders. Most everyone has the best intentions when trying to keep their food plan in order. As we've discussed in detail earlier in the book, life will absolutely get in your way. Not only is it to be expected but I would nearly welcome it. Your strength and your success will depend on not only how you handle this obstacle but how quickly you rebound from it.

Taking a detour from your diet is about as natural as forgetting a common chore. It's bound to happen and it's generally not that serious. The problem lies in the approach that many take: they eat one bad meal and then blow three days out of guilt and disgust with themselves.

This is the portion of the book where I'm giving your power back. Eat the dessert, the burger, the fries, the chips, the pasta, the breadsticks (hopefully not all in one meal). But be painfully honest with yourself about what just happened. You ate it, you likely will NOT un-eat it, and it's time to move on. Step away from the table sir (or ma'am), your damage here is done!

Acknowledge what was done and then get **right back on track**.

Chances are, whatever you cheated on your diet with you probably needed it in some way. Reward yourself mentally with the fact that you have probably been very diligent with your diet up until that point and start thinking about what your next meal back on track will look like. However, what happens if things do spiral completely out of hand and you take a whole weekend to misbehave with your diet?

Nothing happens. Get right back on the plan when Monday rolls around. Will you have gained weight? Maybe. Is it a big deal worth pulling the sky down over? Absolutely not. Chalk it up as a loss and get on with your life. If this book aims to accomplish anything for you, it's that guilt will not guide you. You might have some pangs of it when times get tough (believe me, they will), but you're free to make mistakes, forgive yourself, and push forward.

Just because you had a weak moment(s) does not mean you are a weak person. And just because you struggled to stay on plan does not make you a failure. This circumstance is so common it's nearly laughable. A very popular weight loss program frequently encourages clients to consider their days as purely good or bad. This is a huge mistake!! What ends up happening is that clients consider the days they've starved themselves as the good days because they didn't go over their calorie plan and the days they blew it as bad days.

I'm freeing you from these chains today. Remove them and put your big kid pants back on. Whatever dietary indiscretions you had can generally be very quickly undone. Most clients can undo their luxuries in less than a week after monitoring water intake, fiber intake and getting back to their plan.

If this book accomplishes anything, it's to give you your life back so you can focus on all of the things that matter. Having autonomy over how you handle the missteps is one of the most powerful weapons in your arsenal.

What I will add for most of you who struggle with this is to document the incidents. Write down a few things about the deviation. Date the occurrence. As I'm writing this chapter, I'm only a few days removed from my 40th birthday party. I made the mistake of not really eating very much or drinking very much water throughout the day. I knew there would be a ton of food, desserts, and alcohol at the party so I figured I would save my calories for the event. As it turned out, I was so busy talking with everyone who showed up that I barely ate or drank anything. Not to mention, I was almost completely dehydrated because I didn't have enough water throughout the day.

The next day, I felt like I was hit by a truck. Almost as if I had a nasty hangover without the abundance of alcohol! It took me almost an entire day of increasing my water intake and several small meals (plus a nap), just to get my body to feel normal again. What a wake up call!

Documenting something like this gives not only some clarity to the situation but black-and-white feedback as proof of what happened. Otherwise, it would be easy to let time pass and forget that I did this to myself. While it didn't affect my body weight very much, it did leave me feeling completely out-of-sorts the entire next day. Not a great way to waste a day off from work.

So, use this chapter as your chance to get some foundation for failure. It's ok to fail, normal to fail, and expected that you will fail. Do so willingly and even if you let things get temporarily out of hand, you have new tools to be reasonable with yourself to get things back under control.

Although I've spent a fair amount of time talking about documentation, we'll go into a bit more detail in the next chapter.

Track Or Die

So far, I've mentioned a good deal about documenting things along the way on your journey. I've known a good handful of people who bristle up at the thought of having to write things down. For one, it's inconvenient. Many people don't want to carry around pad and pen and be nestled away somewhere writing down all of the things they've been doing or not doing.

And while I will agree, it can be inconvenient, it's also arguably the most effective way for you to get a grasp on what you've done or how you've felt about it. The good news is, you don't have to do it every day for the rest of your life. You may only need a few days or a few weeks worth of information so you can gain a clearer understanding of your starting point and your evolution throughout your journey.

Many dietitians will ask for a food log from their clients. They're looking for trends, behaviors and other things of note to assess the lifestyles of their clients. If we were to simply go on our own memory, the recollections become vague and muddy at best. Since we have an innate tendency to not want to disappoint others, it's easy to paint our own pictures as a bit rosier than normal. I know some who will cross the line into downright fallacy if given the opportunity. It's not because they intend to lie, it's that the truth can sometimes be just alarming enough to be an embarrassment.

You can take solace in the fact that what you elect to document is really only for your eyes alone. We talked about support systems earlier in the book and there is the chance that you might want to share your journal entries with one of your supports. That is completely up to you. If there is someone in your corner who you feel would be unbiased and constructively critical, you are welcome to use them.

Truth be told, as much as I love discussing food and food behaviors with my clients, I couldn't tell you what I had to eat three days ago at 3pm, or was it 4:30? By the way, did I eat too much of it? Also, there was that bag of chips over on the counter. Did I unconsciously grab a few and forget about it? All of these things should be considered and taken in stride.

Documenting your behaviors is not meant to make you feel bad about yourself. In reality, it's no different than looking at your bank account online. You get black-and-white indisputable data to tell you how much money you have, how much (and for what) you spent, and how you're going to balance the remainder. Tracking what and when you eat is one of the greatest gifts you can give yourself when it comes to what you're trying to do.

If you want to get a greater grasp on how your eating is affecting you, it will be immensely helpful if you can make a note of how these things make you feel. For instance, let's say you have a tendency to skip breakfast. By time you get to your first meal of the day, you could be really hungry. If you trend towards overeating in that first meal, it would be beneficial for you to write something down about it. A journal entry might look something like this:

Thursday, Nov. 19

11:30am-Skipped breakfast today and have had 3 cups of coffee so far. Sat down to eat lunch and ordered a footlong sub instead of a six-inch. The cashier asked me if I wanted to make it a combo with chips, a cookie, and a soft drink. I couldn't resist! I was so hungry! After I ate, I was so stuffed I had trouble catching my breath. Off to conquer the rest of the day!

Now, I'll be honest: I wrote this specifically in a way that would get my attention. It brings a few things to mind.

1) Should I be making a habit of skipping breakfast if my first meal looks like this?

2) Did I really need an extra six inches of a sub when normally the first six is sufficient?

3) Ok, Jason, get a grip. There was no need for chips, cookie and the soft drink!! Surely I have more self control than that!! Plus, I never normally order soft drinks!!

It's this type of self-realization that can spark change.

No need for over-the-top shaming or guilt. I should also note that in typing out that hypothetical journal entry, it took less than two minutes. If I had been writing it down by hand, maybe it might have taken a little bit longer and if I had been typing that info into the note section of my phone, maybe a bit longer as well. Either way, it unveils a lot of things that I might normally forget about if asked to recount it at a later date.

Documenting how you eat gives you the opportunity to come clean and get real. It won't feel normal to do because most people are not in the habit of this type of work. It's almost like unveiling a diary of our deepest darkest secrets. Fortunately, it's not that dramatic.

You can get a lot of eye-opening information to understand how to fix things by just a few days of work. Some people find they want to hold themselves accountable for longer. I would recommend at least one full week. This way you get a clear example of given weekdays and your weekend behaviors.

There are some things you want to be conscious of as well. From a calorie standpoint, not everything as clear as it should be. Many people forget about the creamer and the sugar they use in their coffee. They also lost track of how much salad dressing was on their salad or how much mayonnaise was on their sandwich. Work to be mindful of all of the places where extra calories might be around.

If I was being honest with myself in my journal example, I might also mention how large of a soft drink I ordered and if I put extra cheese or a calorie laden condiment on my sandwich. These things can add up quickly for those looking to find places to cut back on calories.

I'm also trying to set the stage for how important documentation can be when you start implementing the exercise portion of this book. So, what do you say? Ready to start moving?

Phase IV-Action Plan

1.)Determine the best method for gaining control over your eating habits. If you pick the wrong option the first time, try another. Remember there is no absolute wrong way to go but there may be a wrong way at this point in your life.

2.)Give yourself permission to make mistakes. Own up to them, don't deny them and then set yourself back on track. Forgiveness first and then progress.

3.)Document where necessary to hold yourself accountable. This data can be your lifesaver when it comes to being fully aware and conscious of your decisions.

Phase V-Your Fitness

A Template

You're never going to find a shortage of fitness information. The great thing about fitness is: most of what you need to know has been around for a long time. While there may be some new approaches out there to consider, it's safe to say that basically anything you need to do for your exercise regimen has been around longer than you and I have.

I should also take this time to mention that if you have any pre-existing injuries, you need to consult with your doctor first before embarking on any of the plans in this book. If you have the clearance of the professionals, take the time to explain what this book is offering. I am not a doctor and what you will read here does not and should not take the place of what your doctor recommends for you.

I also think that, like food, people over complicate things with fitness. First and foremost, you need consistency. You don't need anything flashy and in many cases you don't need anything expensive. In other words, 20lbs of weight will always be 20lbs of weight. What matters is: can you lift it and how many times?

The average person should probably focus on full-body workouts 2-3 times per week. In addition, if you need to focus on weight loss, you can incorporate more cardio (so you can burn more calories) and if you need to maintain weight or put some mass on, you should incorporate less cardio.

The exercises I'll show you are grouped together based on the primary muscle being worked. Once you have a basic idea of what the exercises look like, you can construct your own workout.

In efforts to keep things as simple as possible but still give you autonomy, we'll be focusing essentially on exercises that work your lower body, upper body (back and chest), with some isolation work (biceps, triceps, shoulders) and core work. You'll pick 6 exercises which incorporate the groups listed above and perform your workouts in that fashion. Beyond that, you can challenge yourself on exercise order and intensity.

For most people, we'll be concentrating on a repetition range of 8-15 reps and 3 sets of exercises. This will give you ample stimulation to see muscle growth and fat loss (in combination with the diet principles in the previous chapter).

Here is your list of exercises to choose from:

Lower Body

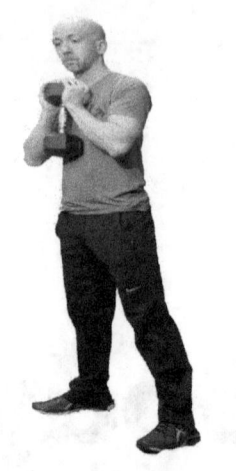

Goblet Squat

Start with a stance that is roughly shoulder width apart. You may need to go wider or narrower depending on your build. You can also flare your toes out 10-20% degrees.

Lower yourself until your legs are about parallel with the floor, then raise back up.

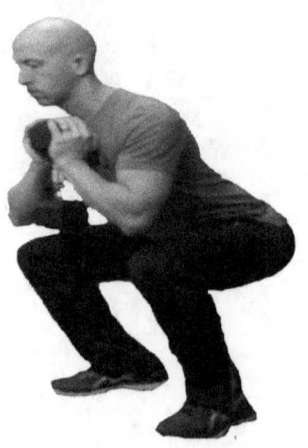

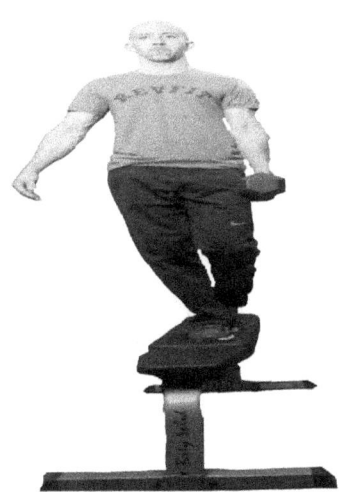

Lateral Step Up
(You can use any raised platform. A step, bench or hard box.)

Drive your weight through the leg that is elevated.

Allow yourself to get centered and balanced at the top and then descend back to the ground.

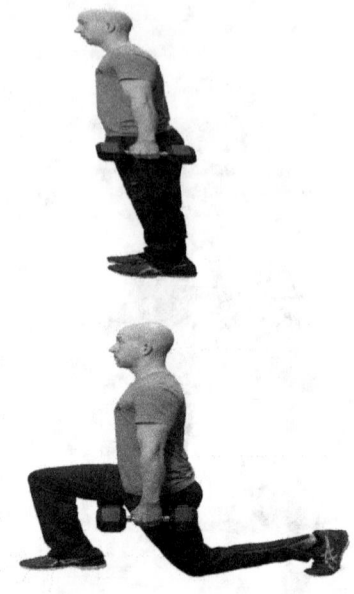

Forward Lunge

Step forward, keeping your back knee just above the ground.

Pause slightly and then return to the standing position.

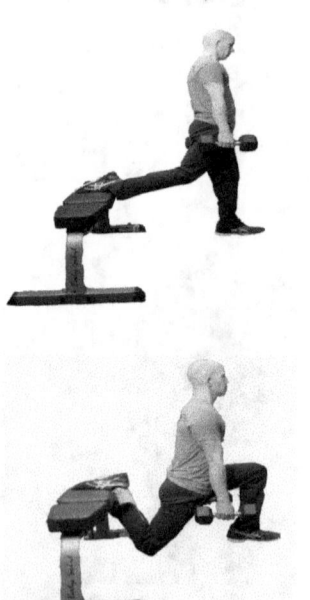

Bulgarian Split Squat

Give yourself ample distance with your front leg so you're not crowding yourself as you descend.

Drop down and pause slightly before standing back up.

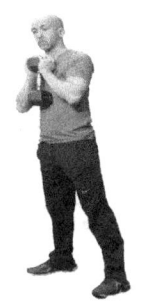

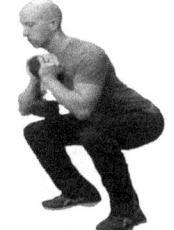

Goblet Squat to Lunge

Start in typical Goblet Squat fashion.

Drop into your squat and then stand back up.

Re-align your legs slightly so you can step forward into your lunge.

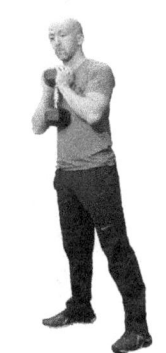

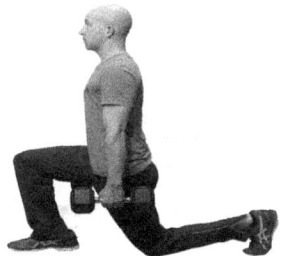

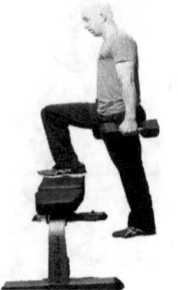

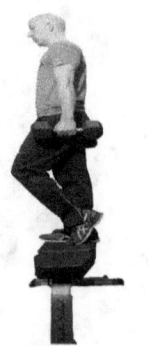

Step-Up

Drive your weight through your

elevated leg.

Pause for a moment at the top before stepping back down.

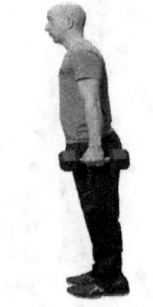

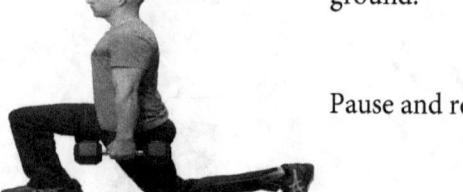

Reverse Lunge

Step back from a standing position. Try to keep your back knee above ground.

Pause and return to standing position.

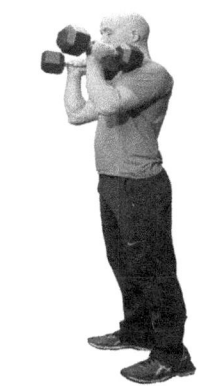

Thruster

Start with dumbbells at shoulder height.

Drop into a squat and "thrust" up with dumbbells finishing overhead.

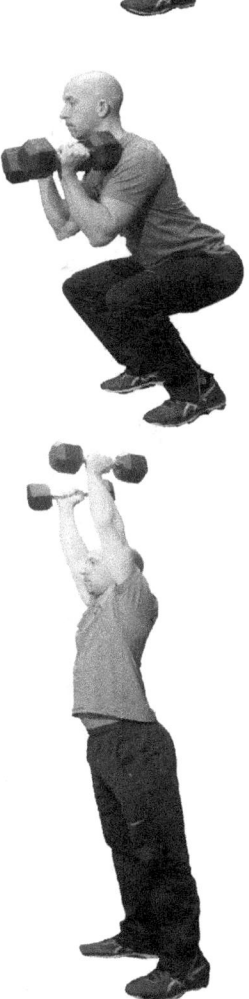

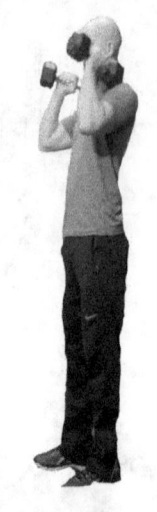

Dumbbell Front Squat

Start with dumbbells at shoulder height.

Descend until legs are about parallel with the ground.

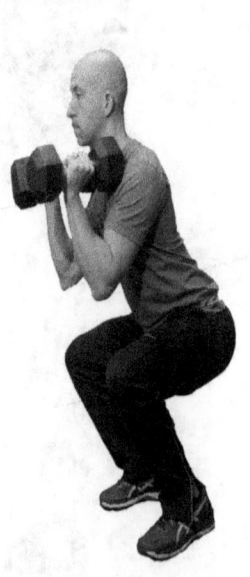

Upper Body
Back

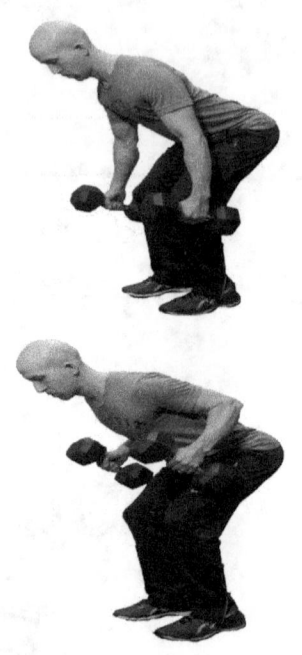

Bent Row

Drive your hips back and keep your lower back from rounding.

Row the dumbbells back keeping elbows close (but not touching) to the sides

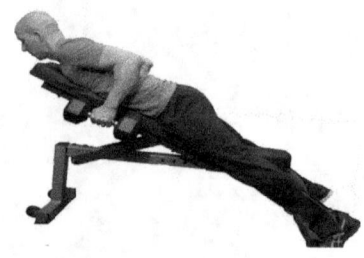

Chest Supported Row

Keep legs extended back behind you and chest pressed firmly into bench.

Row back with a slight pause and slow descent.

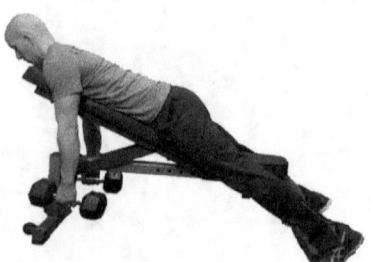

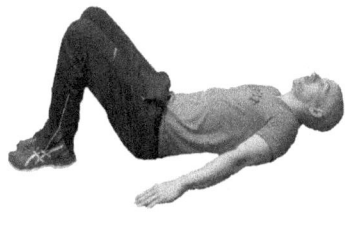

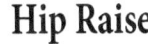

Hip Raise

Squeeze your glutes for 1-2 seconds at the top of the movement.

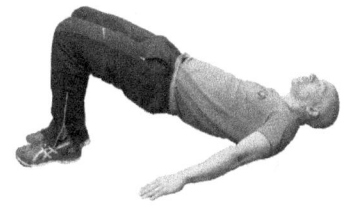

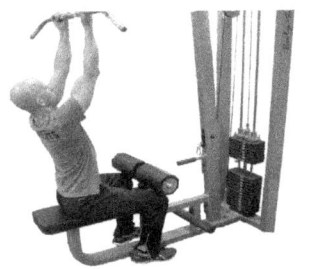

Close-Grip Pulldown

Keep the weight controlled as you pull the weight down to your chest.

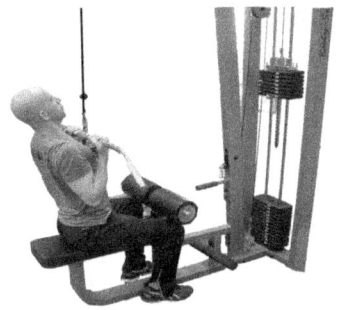

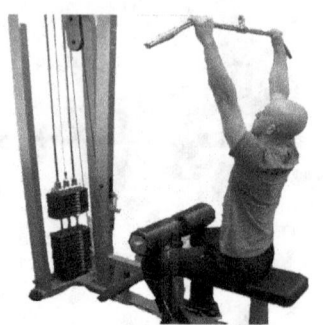

Wide-Grip Pulldown

Keep the weight controlled as you pull the weight down to your chest.

Hold the weight for a slight pause at the bot-tom before raising your arms slowly to com-plete another rep.

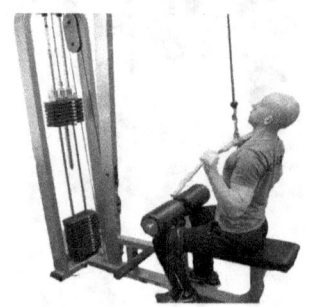

Elevated Hip Raise

Start with your legs at approximately a 90 de-gree angle.

Raise your hips and squeeze your glutes for 1-2 seconds at the top of the movement.

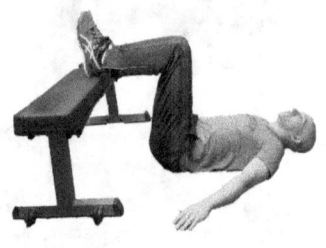

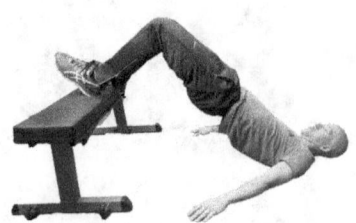

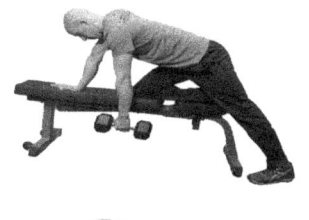

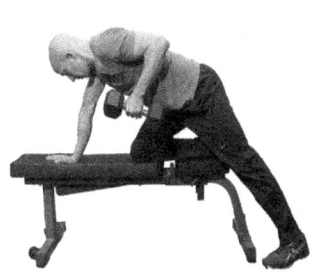

Single-Arm Row

Try to keep your back as flat as possible while rowing.

Resist the temptation to rotate your lower back as you row the weight.

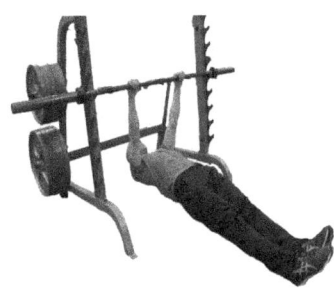

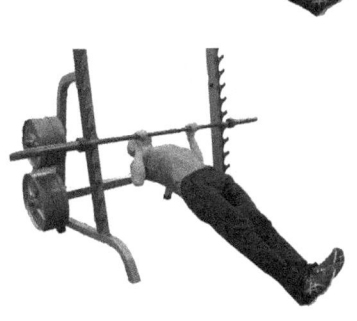

Inverted Row

An easier variation is to bend the knees, flat-ten the feet and raise the hips. This limits the range of motion in this exercise until you can work up to the legs (extended variation in the picture).

Keep your core tight while you pull your body up to the bar.

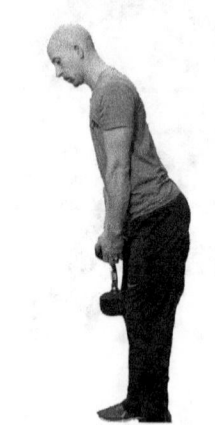

Romanian Deadlift (RDL)

Drive your hips back until your torso is about parallel with the ground.

You should feel a big stretch in your ham-strings (back of your upper leg) when you do this exercise.

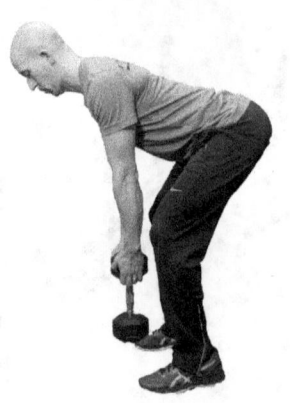

Upper Body
Chest

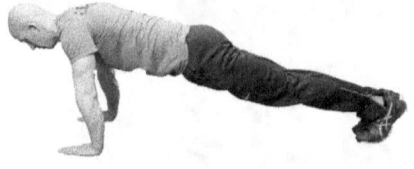

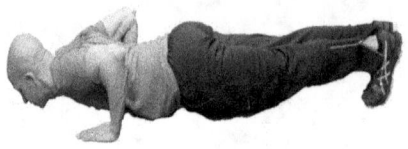

Push-Up

Keep elbows closer to the side as you descend.

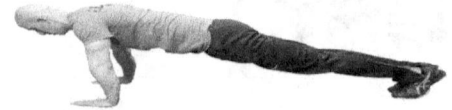

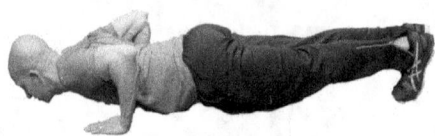

Yoga Push-Up

This is performed almost identical to a stan-dard push-up but you'll allow your hips to pike up at the end of the movement.

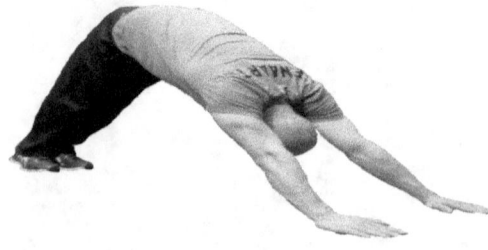

Single-Arm Press

Your opposite arm (the one without the weight) can either be held at the hip or stretched out for variations in core stability

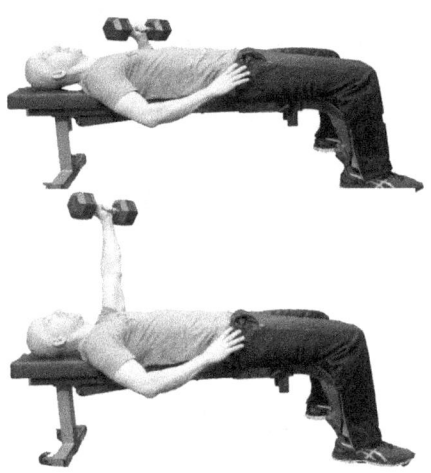

Incline Dumbbell Press

Try to keep elbows closer to the side (with-out touching the side). This should keep you from flaring out too much and imping-ing the shoulder.

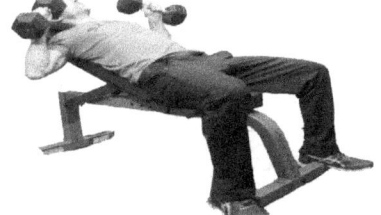

Flat Bench Dumbell Press

This movement is identical to the incline dumbbell press. The only change is the in-cline, which is now flat.

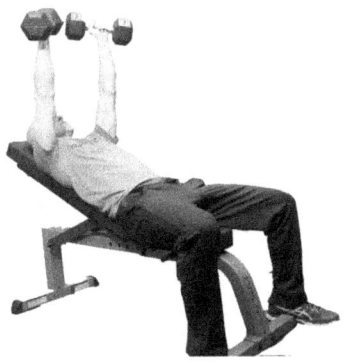

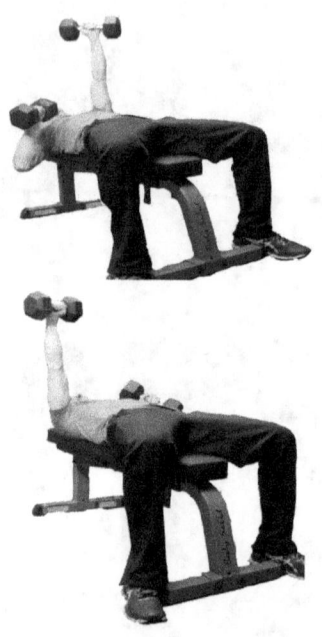

Alternating Dumbbell Press

Alternate the pressing motion in a piston-like fashion from side to side.

Diamond Push-Up

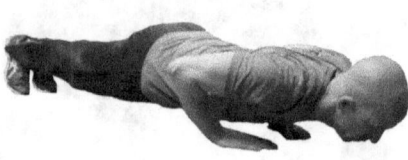

Hands will be placed close together just under the chest.

Elbows will finish close to the rip cage as you descend.

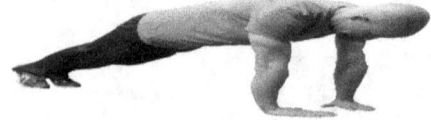

Staggered Push-Up

Allow both elbows to bend so you
still get appropriate range of
motion out of your arms. If this
exercise is too difficult as show, you
can perform it with knees down.

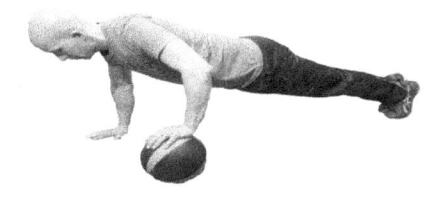

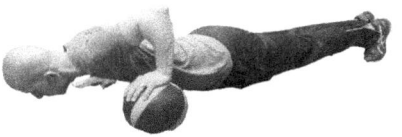

Floor Press

Keep legs extended out (not bent).

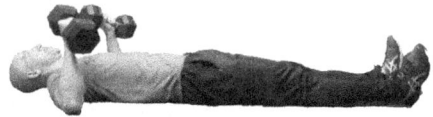

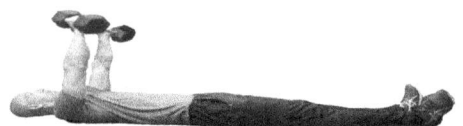

Isolation:
Bicep, Tricep and Shoulder

(Pick TWO per Workout)

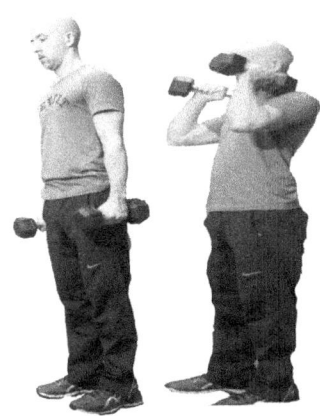

Hammer Curl

Start with a neutral grip (palms facing the sides)

Curl the weight straight up in that grip

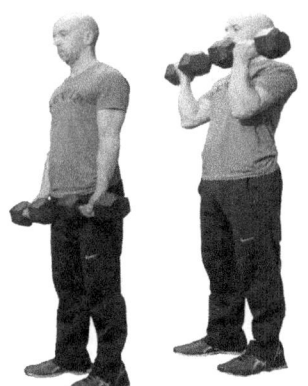

Front Curl

Start with palms facing out

Curl the weight straight up, elbows close to the sides.

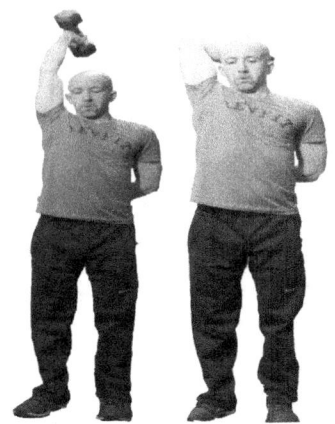

Single-Arm Overhead Extension

Try to keep your arm close to your ear during this movement. Due to the shoulder mobility of certain individuals, you may not look identi-cal to the picture.

Neutral Overhead Press

Resist the temptation to arch the lower back on this exercise.

Keep the core stable as you press the weight overhead.

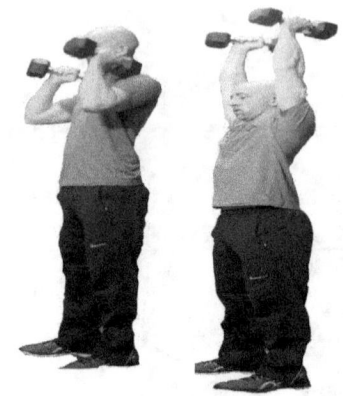

Lying Extension

Note the starting angle of the upper arms in this exercise.

Try not to throw the arms forward as you bring the weight back up. This will take the tension off your triceps here.

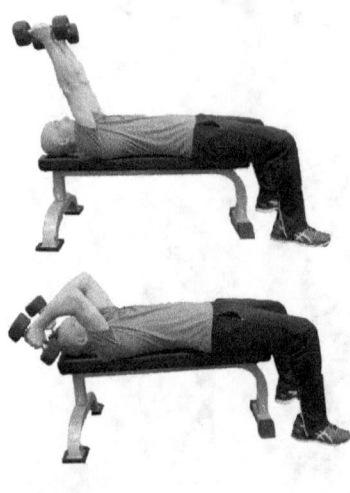

Twisting Curl

Start with a neutral grip (palms facing sides).

Twist the weight up as you curl allowing the palms to face the shoulders at the top.

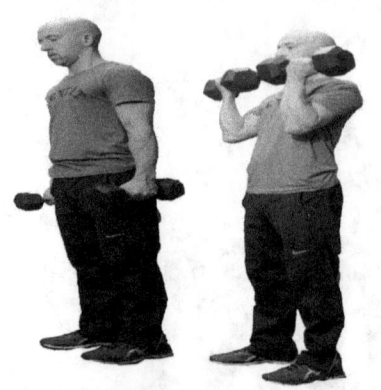

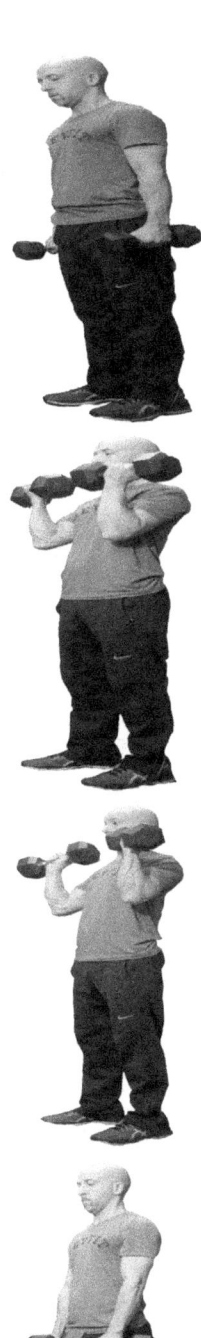

Zottman Curl

Start with a neutral grip (palms facing sides).

Twist the weight up as you curl allowing the palms to face the shoulders at the top.

Turn the palms out and slowly let the dumb-bells descend down.

At the bottom of the movement the palms should be facing the body.

Overhead Extension

Resist the temptation to let the back arch ex-cessively on this exercise.

Keep the weight controlled during the entire movement.

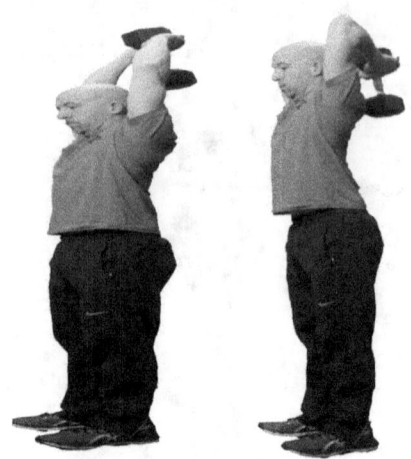

Cable Pressdowns

Hold your chest high during this movement without letting the shoulders round forward.

Split the cable out to the sides at the bottom of the movement.

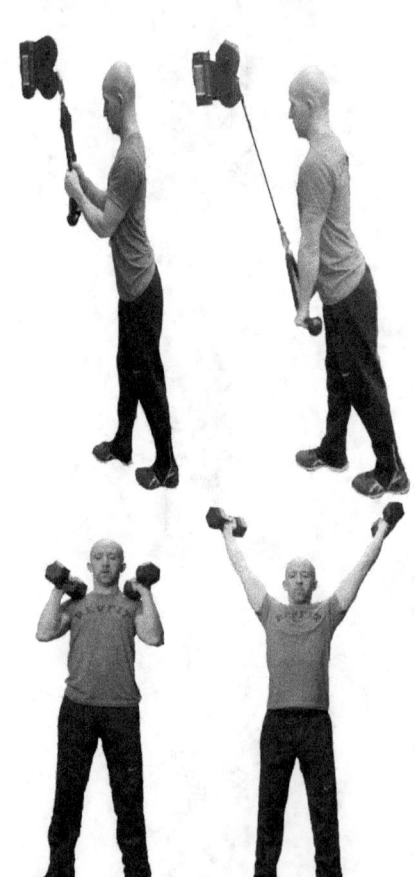

Y Press

Start conservatively with the weight on this exercise to get a better feeling for how the shoulder will respond.

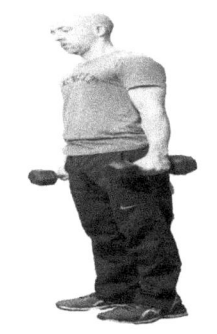

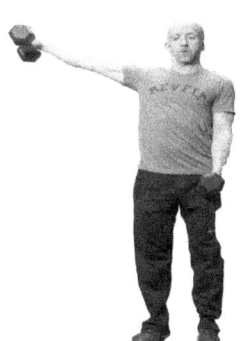

Alternating Lat Raise

Don't swing the weight during this

movement.

Keep the raising and lowering under
control at all times.

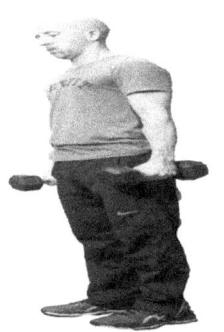

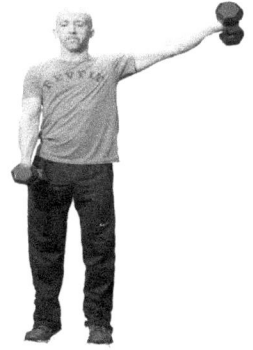

Core

Plank

Brace your core (stomach and lower back) and glutes during this exercise.

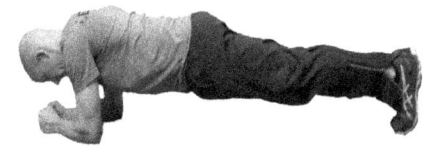

Side Plank

Brace your core (stomach and lower back) and glutes during this exercise.

Make sure feet, hips and back are in alignment.

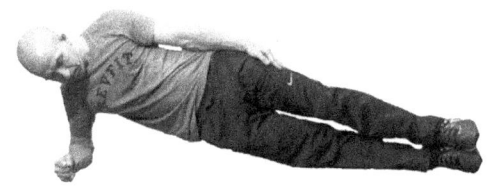

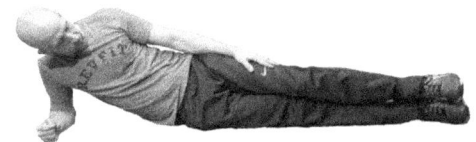

Side Dip Plank

Start in a side plank position

Allow the lower hip to dip down towards the floor then raise back up.

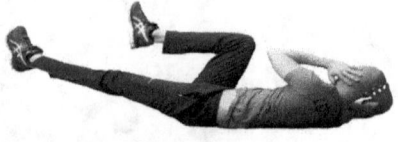

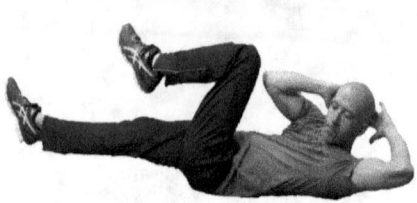

Bicycle

Keep this movement controlled so you don't aggravate
your lower back.

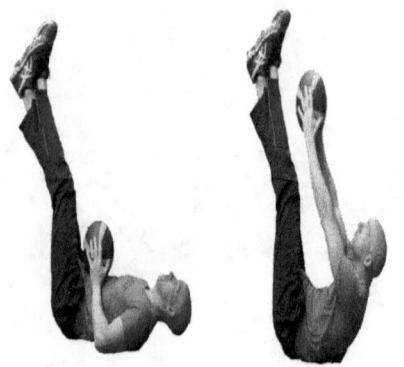

Medicine Ball Toe Touch

Press the ball from the belly not from the chest.

Try to keep legs stationary.

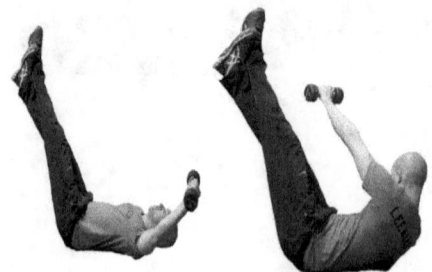

Cross Lateral Toe Touch

Bring the weight across the body and outside the opposite leg.

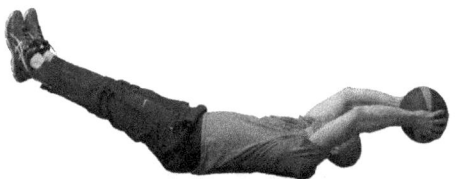

Single-Leg Tuck

Keep this movement controlled so you don't aggravate your lower back.

Alternate sides during this exercise

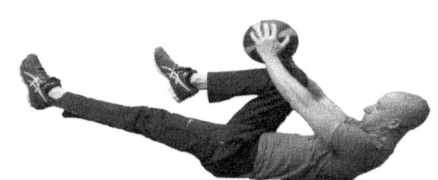

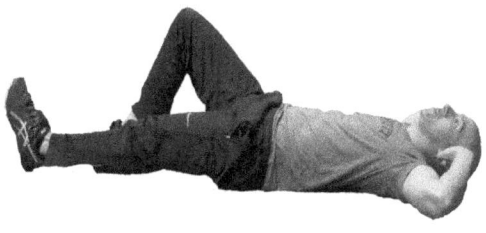

McGill Curl Up

This is a very isolated exercise. Keep the core pressed down at all times. When doing this exercise for time (30 seconds each side), make sure you alternate leg position.

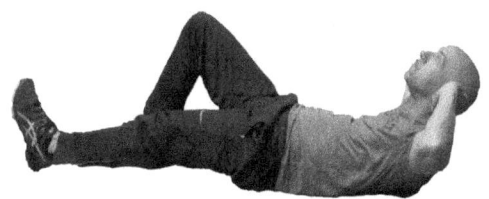

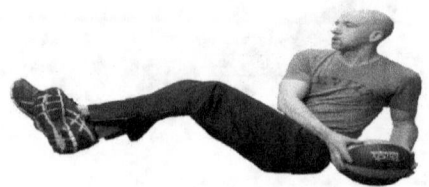

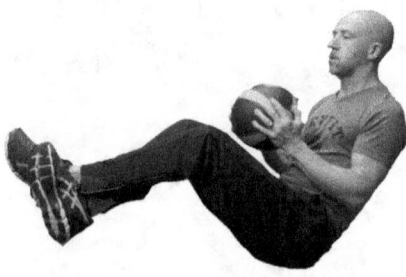

Russian Twist

You can perform this exercise with feet up or down.

Feet up will increase the difficulty.

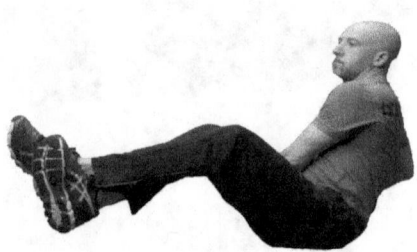

For any exercise excluding the core work, you'll pick a weight that allows you to work within an 8-15 rep range. If you can't get within that range, you've gone to heavy. By comparison, if you can hit 15 reps and you still have plenty of energy to do more, you've gone too light.

In case you haven't thought about it yet, this is where I'm going to be redundant and say that now is definitely the time when you'll want a journal of what you're doing. You need proof of the order you worked in so you can see where you've gone up in weights or reps. Ultimately, you have to see progress in one or the other.

Now, depending on your age and starting point when reading this, you may not be as concerned about getting stronger. For certain people, just moving and getting their bodies and muscles stimulated will be sufficient. I encourage you to get as strong as you can relative to your goals. Basically, we're all chasing Father Time so your goal (in as much as I can influence it) is to build and maintain all of that precious muscle before you get to the point where you can't. And if you're a woman reading this book, that doesn't mean I'm asking you to get bulky. Simply put, you don't produce enough testosterone for that to be an issue.

From the list of exercises, pick one exercise from each group to design your first workout. In the core work, aim for time rather than repetition. I normally time the core work between 30-60 seconds.

Here's what a sample workout should look like assuming we take the first exercises out of each group. Note the first number is the amount of weight and the second number is the amount of reps performed:

Goblet Squat 20 x 12/25 x 12/30 x 12

Bent Row 15 x 12/20 x 12/25 x 12

Push Up 15/15/12

Front Raise 10 x 12/10 x 12/10 x 12

Hammer Curl 15 x 15/15 x 15/ 15 x 15

Plank 30 secs/30 secs/30 secs

There are several things to keep in mind when looking at this sample workout. If you need more recovery between exercises, you can simply go through each exercise once until you've completed all six exercises. That would be one set. Then repeat the set in that order once or twice more. If you want more intensity you can limit your recovery between exercises by changing the order slightly.

One option is to take two exercises at a time and do them back-to-back until you've completed 3 sets. It would look like this:

Goblet Squat (20 x 12), Bent Row (15 x 12)

Take a 30-90 second break

Goblet Squat (25 x 12), Bent Row (20 x 12)

Take a 30-90 second break

Goblet Squat (30 x 12), Bent Row (25 x 12)

Take a 30-90 second break

Once you've completed these exercises in this order, you can move on to the next two exercises and complete them in the same way. After you've done this for all six exercises, your workout would be done for the day.

A third option (the most intense), would be to complete all three sets of a given exercise in a row. So, you would perform the Goblet Squat three times in a row with a 30-90 second break in between each set. When you've completed the third set, you would move on to the Bent Row and repeat.

By limiting your recovery between exercises and keeping your recovery time to a minimum, you're raising the intensity of the exercise. These simple variations will keep your muscles stimulated and responding appropriately.

My recommendation is to try each variation as you gain comfort with the format. It's also important to note that you should be constantly searching for different ways to chart progress.

For instance, if you had been working on your Goblet Squat for several weeks, a few different things should be happening: you should be moving up in weight, reps or sets. Progress will not always be linear and you may find that you're stuck at a given weight for an indefinite amount of time. You can still find ways to push your body past the plateau by aiming for 15 reps instead of 12 or by adding a fourth set when your body has been accustomed to only three.

Assuming that you are being diligent with your

journal in tracking your exercises, you will have the indisputable data showing how you've progressed.

As far as your cardiovascular work is concerned, I want you to take a somewhat simple approach. Do as much as you can without wearing yourself out but still allowing ample recovery from your strength work. Remember that building muscle helps you burn calories more efficiently. While cardio work can assist in calorie burning, it can also work against your ability to build muscle. Rather than give you an all-or-nothing approach, I want you to do the cardio that works best for your body while still giving you plenty in the tank for your strength workouts.

If you want to start your journey by walking a couple of times a week first and then adding in your strength work, great! If you prefer to lift weights first and then add in the cardio, this too is great. There is no absolute wrong but you will find out what works best for you rather quickly. Some days will lend themselves to slower and longer bouts of cardio (easier to recover from) and some days will be better for shorter and more intense work. If your food plan is on point and you've found the right eating approach for your lifestyle, the results you want will come.

Think In the Gray

Like I mentioned in the diet section, I can't encourage you enough to allow your thinking to reside somewhere on the inside of the black and white of exercise. That's why I want you to work within the parameters of your exercise journey but without allowing yourself to think it's an all or nothing approach. It's not. Look anywhere around you for exercise options and you'll find more choices than you'll know what to do with: group training, yoga, pilates, CrossFit, private and semi-private personal training, spinning, and more.

I can assure you there will be no shortage of options either. Some things may cycle in and out of vogue but the general recommendation remains roughly the same: lift weights to stimulate your muscles and sculpt your body, do more (or less) cardio depending on your respective goals for conditioning and heart health, and constantly find ways to challenge yourself.

Remember, too, that not every workout will be a great one. Some days will be awesome and you'll feel like previously heavy weights are moving with ease. By the same token, there will be other days when light weights will feel like the heaviest you've ever lifted. Listen to your body and be somewhat conservative when pushing yourself.

If you were embarking on a career as a competitive powerlifter or an ultra-endurance athlete, my advice would be very different. Chances are, you're not reading this book if those are your aspirations. Those individuals have to continue to push themselves outside of the realm of the average person. It's not a right or wrong, it's just the path they've elected to follow and the mindset changes.

When it comes to the way you should approach your exercise regimen, one of the most important principles you can learn is auto-regulation. This is simply the ability to understand how your body and mind are feeling on a given day, and pushing (or pulling back) accordingly. If the workout calls for 12 reps of a given exercise and you're not firing on all cylinders, you have a couple of options: push it for the 12 reps just to hit the number or scale it back and focus more on quality of rep over quantity. As you might expect, quality should always trump quantity. If you listen to your body, you stand less chance of injury and can attack your workout more effectively when you're feeling up to speed. This also goes for people who are considering working out when they're under the weather.

Ultimately, I want you to have flexibility with the way you train. This way you can train indefinitely with as few setbacks as possible. I should say as well, there is always a risk of injury when exercising. I've had my share and if they taught me nothing else, it was to listen more carefully to my body and correct the deficiencies. I also don't want anyone to feel forced into a certain fitness philosophy. Some people love to run, others love to use an elliptical or swim. Experiment and find the activity that gets you closer to your goal and keeps you as consistent as possible with your training plan.

When you find that particular activity, I would also encourage you to go the extra step, and where applicable, find someone who can train you to be better. For instance, if you enjoy running, it would be beneficial to find a running coach or crew who can help you better understand your gait and body mechanics while running. This will not only help you become more efficient but also further from injury.

While I'm on the subject of running, I make this suggestion: get fitted for shoes. I've seen many clients train in the same shoes they would mow their lawns in. While I can appreciate comfort just as much as the next person, you'll be amazed at how a properly fitted pair of shoes can affect your ability to run.

That being said, many running shoes have considerable cushion in the heels. While this can be great for running, it might be problematic for lifting weights. The cushion can present too much instability with exercises like squats and lunges. These days, "minimalist" shoes can provide ample support while training. While this can potentially raise the cost for partaking in both activities, having shoes dedicated for running and shoes dedicated for lifting weights can save you and your joints a lot of anguish.

Phase V-Action Plan

1.) If you haven't done so already, you'll need to purchase a notebook to track your workouts. An inexpensive composition notebook will suffice. Document each of your workouts here.

2.) Ideally, you'll pick one exercise from each major group (two from the isolation section) and design your workout. Feel free to use as much or as little variation from the selections as you like.

3.) Add more cardio work if you need to lose body fat, do less cardio work if you are already at maintenance or are using this template to add muscle mass.

4.) The sky is the limit with your exercise design. You do want variation but not so much variation that you can't get a reasonable outlook on how you've progressed. I would recommend no more than 18 different exercises over the course of one month. You can change exercises from month to month so you see more variety in your program.

Phase VI-Your Goals

How Does It Change?

If you've read many self-help or motivational books, goal setting is one of the biggest signs of success. Countless books talk about the importance of writing down your goals in all variety of ways to have a clearer picture of what you want to accomplish. I have to agree that it is really a big deal. However, the manner in which you do it will be different per individual.

Some people need short-term and long-term goals. Some need daily goals. I've heard of people who write down 3-5 goals on a small sheet of paper and look at it every day to make sure they're mentally focused on what they're aiming for. All of these tactics work. Like I've become somewhat redundant in emphasizing throughout the book, you have to find what works best for you. Assuming that one way and only one way will work is asking for trouble.

And as important as goals are, the process towards reaching them is equally important. Not only should you be clear about where you want to be, but you should have a concept of what steps you'll need to take to get there. For instance, let's say you want to save money for a vacation. Perhaps you've done the due diligence to find out your vacation will cost $5000. Assuming that you won't be charging the expense on credit cards, how will you come up with the money? Will you work more hours at your current job? Will you pick up a part-time job? What about paying off certain debts so you can have some money freed up to put towards your vacation. These are some simple ways of looking at how you'll reach your goals.

But this book isn't as much about financial goals. It's more about the goals you have for your lifestyle. How much do you want to weigh? What pant size do you want to comfortably fit into? How strong do you want to be? Do you want to run a marathon?

Once you've determined those goals, you have to ask yourself what you're willing to compromise or change to get there. One thing is for sure, wherever you are right now, change will have to take place to get you closer to your goals. But the other purpose for this chapter is to prepare you for a common occurrence with goals and reaching them that many people don't consider. What if the goals change along the way?

Let's say you want to lose 40lbs. Assuming that you stay mostly on track with your diet and exercise and you've followed most of the tips I've offered in this book, you're looking at somewhere between 20-40 weeks of effort. 20 weeks is between 4-5 months. 40 weeks is 10 months. When you look at that timeline, how do you see this affecting you? Are you going to start shooting for your goal around the holidays the last few months of the year? If so, how hard will it be for you to stay on track? Or are you going to start over the summer when the weather is nice and you're able to do more outside?

Another thing to consider is: What if 40lbs is too much to ask? Maybe you're like some of the clients who come in to see me, their body has changed from years of medications, changes in hormones and stress levels, and weight that has fluctuated wildly through pregnancies, etc. What if your body could comfortably thrive and maintain at a loss of 25lbs?

These are the questions you'll need to consider if you want long-term success. So many people get focused on one goal without giving themselves the flexibility to meet somewhere in the middle. Your body will naturally want to find that happy medium and balanced state, otherwise referred to as homeostasis. That's why, over the years, I've found several people who can lose massive amounts of weight with little resistance and others who have to kick, scrape and claw their way to lose 15lbs.

I will also say this, if you're only 10-15lbs away from where you really want to be, you don't have a lot of room for error. Your dietary and exercise diligence has to be nearly spot on with as few luxuries as possible.

So, while your goals are immensely important because they can keep you focused, you'll also want to be aware of how things may ebb and flow along the way. Be understanding to the fact that wherever you are in your life right now, what you once could do may take considerably more effort than what you had bargained for. It doesn't make things bad or good, it just means you have to listen appropriately to everything that has an effect: your mindset, your environment, your support system, your diet, and your exercise to see what has to be modified or tweaked along the way for the best end result.

Most importantly, as much as we all want change AND results RIGHT NOW, it really isn't the reality of our situations. Change is hard. Results can be misleading. Focus on every step of your journey but realize where your body and your mind need more attention.

Allow the (R)evolution

I feel as if I've covered a lot with you in a fairly short amount of time. It was my goal with this book to present you with the things my clients struggled with the most and what ultimately led to them being successful. I also used these same principles to overcome my own adversities in life.

If you've been able to act on what you've read so far, I commend you. There are so many changes to consider in this book and not all of them will stick for all people. You may even need to read this book a couple of times to let some of the concepts and strategies sink in. Not because they're complex but because you'll want to be clear on how to implement each into your life.

I've been very blessed with the privilege of seeing many little miracles happen with my clients. When they started to add up, I knew we were on to something special and I had to share it with more people. Maybe there are things that you've read here that are new to you but, hopefully, I presented them in a light where they make more sense and seem more possible for you.

The clients of mine who have seen the most success have embraced these changes and taken control over their lives and their bodies. Many have seen such drastic change that their personal and professional lives improved as well. Taken in scope, if you take care of your body and mind, those who are closest to you get to be beneficiaries as well. Next thing you know, your progress becomes infectious and others will want to know what you've done to transform.

So, with this no-nonsense approach I want you to constantly be in a state of allowing the changes to continue. Your life will always have its respective challenges. There will always be things that can deter you from where you want to be. If you're clear on your purpose and you've worked to surround yourself with the right influence and appropriate changes, you will continue to see the results you deserve.

Expect resistance, anticipate the struggle, and push forward. Constantly strive for ways to add challenge to your routines. Stay just outside of your comfort zone at all times. You deserve all the good you want to accomplish. Earn it and stay driven.

The Revolution Is You.

ABOUT THE AUTHOR

Jason Leenaarts is the owner of Revolution Fitness and Therapy. He started the business in 2009 with the aim of giving balance back to busy people who needed exercise and nutrition to help them realize their goals. Since then, he has trained hundreds of people to maximize their potential. Jason is certified as an Elite I Trainer through ISSA and is a Level 1 Coach through Precision Nutrition.

www.ingramcontent.com/pod-product-compliance
Lightning Source LLC
Chambersburg PA
CBHW072046280526
45788CB00006B/2205